Recent Advances in Medical Statistics

Edited by Cruz Vargas-De-León

Published in London, United Kingdom

Recent Advances in Medical Statistics
http://dx.doi.org/10.5772/intechopen.94647
Edited by Cruz Vargas-De-León

Contributors
Keumhee Chough Carriere, Weng Kee Wong, Yin Li, Su Hwan Kim, Manuel Solís-Navarro, Susana Guadalupe Guzmán-Aquino, Jazmín García-Machorro, María Guzmán-Martínez, Eduardo Pérez-Castro, Ramón Reyes-Carreto, Rocio Acosta-Pech, Flaviano Godinez-Jaimes, Irene Lena Hudson, Paulo Tadeu Meira e Silva de Oliveira, Ainura Tursunalieva, J. Geoffrey Chase, Cruz Vargas-De-León, Edilberta Tino-Salgado, Norma Samanta Romero-Castro, Salvador Reyes-Fernández, Victor Othon Serna-Radilla

First published in London, United Kingdom, 2022 by IntechOpen
IntechOpen is the global imprint of INTECHOPEN LIMITED, registered in England and Wales, registration number: 11086078, 5 Princes Gate Court, London, SW7 2QJ, United Kingdom

British Library Cataloguing-in-Publication Data
A catalogue record for this book is available from the British Library

Additional hard and PDF copies can be obtained from orders@intechopen.com

Recent Advances in Medical Statistics
Edited by Cruz Vargas-De-León
p. cm.
Print ISBN 978-1-80356-077-9
Online ISBN 978-1-80356-078-6
eBook (PDF) ISBN 978-1-80356-079-3

Meet the editor

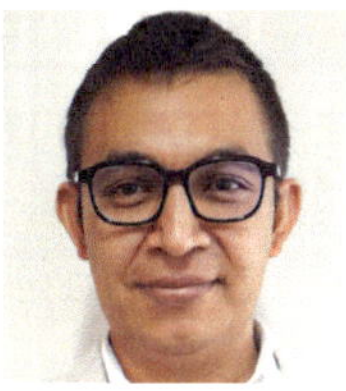

Cruz Vargas-De-León is a Researcher in Medical Sciences at the Hospital Juárez de Mexico in Magdalena De Las Salinas, Mexico City. He has a bachelor's degree in mathematics (statistics), a master's degree in health sciences, a master's degree in complexity sciences, and a Ph.D. in health sciences. His research interests are biostatistical and biomathematical modeling for health. He has published more than 60 articles, 40 of them in high-impact journals and JCR indexed. He has participated in the validation of surveys, randomized controlled trials, systematic reviews and meta-analyses, the construction of indices in medicine, the identification of immunological biomarkers in cancer and epidemiological studies, and the estimation of parameters of differential equation models. He received a certificate for highly cited research in *Mathematical Biosciences* (2016, Elsevier) and was awarded the Guillermo Soberón Guerrero State Award for Merit in Science and Technology (2016). His biography appeared in Marquis *Who's Who in the World*, Issue 30 (2013). Two of his articles received "excellent paper" awards from the National Program for Research Evaluation (2011-2014) in Italy. He has been a member of the National System of Researchers of Mexico's National Council of Science and Technology since 2015.

Contents

Preface

Statistics is one of the most widely applied branches of mathematics in science. Among the advances in complex statistical methods through which statisticians can provide a greater understanding of complex processes and mechanisms are applications in medical sciences and health sciences, including generalized linear models, structural equation models, spatial statistical models, statistical methods for clinical trials, Copula models, multi-state models for the analysis of time-to-event data, and multilevel models.

This book is divided into three sections: biostatistical modeling, spatial statistics, and clinical trials. Section 1, 'Biostatistical Modelling', contains five contributions. Chapter 1 proposes the use of binary and ordinal logistic regression techniques to calculate the risk probability for different disabilities (visual, hearing, physical, and intellectual). The author uses criteria such as Akaike Information Criterion (AIC) and Bayesian Information Criterion (BIC) to perform a selection of variables and selected models. Chapter 2 is a detailed introduction to structural equation models in medicine and health sciences and provides an example of their use in the 'red code' process. Chapter 3 illustrates the use of the empirical transition matrix and multi-state modeling to develop advanced optimal infusion controllers and to help nurses encode agitation-sedation scores. Chapter 4 introduces Copula models to capture non-linear dependence and establish the presence of lower- and/or upper-tail dependence between the nurse's agitation-sedation rating and the automated sedation dose. Chapter 5 discusses the use of multilevel models in dental research when the response variable is numerical and shows how the bottom-up strategy can be adapted to specify a multilevel model in the Bayesian approach.

Section 2, 'Spatial Statistics', consists of two chapters. Chapter 6 presents spatial models used in epidemiology to predict infectious and non-infectious diseases occurring in a region: generalized linear spatial models, spatial survival models and spatial generalized extreme value models. Chapter 7 demonstrates the application of spatial statistics with the implementation of a generalized linear spatial model for the prediction of dengue disease in the state of Chiapas.

Section 3, 'Clinical Trials' contains two chapters. Chapter 8 discusses practical and near-optimal designs for clinical trials and reviews the strategy of incorporating multiple objectives while advocating a regression-type estimation approach via the generalized estimating equations method. The authors show that the adaptive allocation scheme successfully constructs designs of the desired efficiency, illustrated by practical two- and three-period designs. Chapter 9 reviews fundamental ideas, models, and the construction of optimal designs for N-of-1 trials, and discusses how they may be aggregated to estimate treatment effects for the average patient.

I would like to express my thanks to Karla Skuliber for her support throughout the editorial process of this book.

Cruz Vargas-De-León
Professor,
División de Investigación,
Hospital Juárez de México,
Ciudad de México, México

Section 1

Biostatistical Modelling

Chapter 1

Logistic Regression: Risk Question for Disabled People

Paulo Tadeu Meira e Silva de Oliveira

Abstract

All over the world, since ancient times, disabled people have always had worse health, education, economical participation, and higher poverty rate compared to non-disabled people. For disabled people to achieve better and more lasting prospects, these people must be empowered and seek to eliminate barriers that prevent them from participating and being included in the community, having access to quality education, finding decent work, and having their voices heard. In statistical terms, a useful alternative that can serve as support and monitoring of public policies in this area is to propose, for continuous use, the risk index called risk index for disabled people (long-term physical, hearing, intellectual, or sensory), which consists of evaluating which factors are associated with this risk, as well its intensity and direction of each of these factors, generating a final score that can be ordered or classified, according to non-disabled person probability became disabled person. In the Brazilian case, we propose the use of binary and ordinal logistic regression techniques to select the most significant factors using criteria such as AIC and BIC and calculate the risk probability for different disabilities (visual, hearing, physical, and intellectual) for the dataset. Sample composed of 20,800,804 respondents to the 2010 IBGE Census Complete Questionnaire.

Keywords: disabled people, disability risk, variable selection, model selection, stereotype ordinal logistic regression

1. Introduction

According to the World Health Organization (WHO) in 2010, it is estimated that more than one billion people from all over the world, representing about 15% of the world population and in the case of Brazil, according to the Geography Brazilian Institute (IBGE) in 2010, it is estimated that 45.6 million people, equivalent to approximately 23.9% of the Brazilian population, live with some type of disability. In general, disabled people have worse health prospects, educational, economical participation, and a higher rate of poverty compared to non-disabled people.

Disabled people make up a group of excluded people who have always aroused feelings that range from repulsion to extreme pity and have even been considered less human or lacking in humanity. Currently, within the scope of social and educational inclusion policies, they have become the target of affirmative actions, which seek to guarantee their rights in various aspects of life in society [1, 2].

It is believed that the low working conditions of disabled people are due to situations such as: difficulty in accessing education, inadequate infrastructure, prejudice, little knowledge, and better accessibility conditions on the part of schools and companies that make these people have a lower education, which makes it difficult to enter the formal job market [3].

In order for disabled people to achieve better and more lasting prospects, it is necessary to empower them and remove barriers that prevent them from participating in the community, accessing quality education, finding decent work, and having their voices heard [4].

To better assess the needs of disabled people, it is necessary to describe this group of people to know the answers to questions such as: How many are there? Where they live? How do you live? What implications does disability have on these people's access to all the different human services in an autonomous and comprehensive way? In short, how can disability influence the life quality of these people?

In statistical terms, it shows the existence of few formal studies, among which the data obtained through censuses stand out, allowing questions such as: How are disabled people distributed across the country? How to assess the access of disabled people to the different services mentioned earlier? How is the evolution of disabled people when comparing them with those without disabilities? What would be the variables that most contribute to cases of disability? How do disabled people compare to people without disabilities? Answering these and other questions can contribute to better support for these people so that they can be better assisted and resources to be better managed and optimized by public policy actions in this area.

Statistically, a useful alternative to assist in the monitoring of public policies in this area is the risk index, which consists of evaluating which factors are most impacting for this risk, as well as its intensity and direction, generating a score that can be ordered or classified according to the probability of people becoming disabled. In the case of this work, we propose the use of techniques such as binary and ordinal logistic regression to select the most significant factors by applying criteria such as binary and ordinal logistic regression to select the most significant factors by applying criteria such as Akaike Information Criterion (AIC), Bayesian Information Criterion (BIC), and Deviation Information Criterion (DIC) and calculate the risk probability for the different disabilities (vision, hearing, movement, and intellectual) for the sample dataset composed of 20,800,804 respondents of the Complete Questionnaire of the IBGE 2010 Census by state, region, and country.

In a previous work [1], we considered as response variable, the different disabilities, and the existence of at least one disability as binary variable, that is, whether a given individual is or is not a disability person. In this work, we are considering the different deficiencies, incorporating their different degrees of severity and number of deficiencies as ordinal response variable, which allows better quality in terms of information and fit in the model.

In Section 2, we present an introduction to the problem, we establish and characterize the variables to be used, the stereotyped ordinal logistic model, selection of variables such as the Wald test, and models using the AIC, BIC, and DIC criteria, and we define the risk of disability for different degrees of severity "cannot at all," "can, but with great difficulty" and "can, but with a little difficulty" for visual, hearing and physical disability, and, in the case of intellectual disability, it was proposed the following levels the use of the risk "has" or "does not have" intellectual disability. In Section 3, we present results and discussions; and, in Section 4, we present conclusions and suggestions for future work.

2. Materials and methods

2.1 Motivation

For better inclusion of disabled people, it is important to know what are the factors that most impact the conditions of these people. In this work, we propose the adjustment of stereotyped ordinal logistic models to incorporate the most significant factors using AIC, BIC, and DIC as selection criteria, creation and determination of the risk of deficiency for a set of sample data of the respondents of the Complete Questionnaire of the 2010 IBGE Census.

2.2 Data description

The variables were obtained directly from the questionnaire applied to the dataset of the sample that responded to the Complete Questionnaire and can be found on the website www.ibge.gov.br in the 2010 Census, sample, and microdata with more details about its description in Oliveira [1].

2.3 Ordinal logistic regression

A good number of the variables used in the social sciences and humanities are ordinal. Often, the dependent variable takes discrete values, or sortable categories, but the distance between them is neither known nor constant. For example, in epidemiological studies, the level of severity of visual, hearing, or physical is set out in the 2010 Demographic Census Sample Questionnaire, which can be classified as ¨*can not at all,*¨ ¨*he succeeds, but with great difficulty,*¨ ¨*can, but with a little difficulty*,¨ and, finally, "*no problem*" to hear, see, or get around. In the case of intellectual disability, it is divided into ¨*has*¨ or ¨*has not.*¨

Among possible adjustment models for ordinal logistic regression, the following ones stand out: proportional probability model, more suitable for interpretation when the response variable is continuous and has been categorized; continuous ratio model, suitable in situations where there is specific interest in a particular category of the response variable; partial proportional probability model that allows to moderate covariates with the assumption of proportional probabilities, and for other variables in which this assumption is not satisfied, specific parameters that vary for the different categories compared and an extension of the proportional probability model are included in the model; and finally, stereotype model, proposed by [5–7]) used in situations where the response variable is ordinal, which is not a discrete version of some continuous variable that was considered in this research.

For this work, we have response variables: visual, hearing, physical, and intellectual disabilities, which are ordinal variables. In view of this, we adopted the stereotyped model in this work.

2.3.1 Stereotype model specification

Imagine that the dependent variable consists of J categories ($m = 1, \ldots, J$) and consider K predictors ($J = 1, \ldots, K$). The stereotype ordinal model is defined at an early stage with the multinomial regression model to which the condition is added $\beta_{m|J} \equiv \varphi_m \hat{\beta}$, where J is the reference category, that is, we have that the multinomial regression model is given by:

$$\text{Prob}(\text{y} = \text{m}|\text{x}) = \frac{\exp\left(\beta'_{m|J}x\right)}{\sum_{j=1}^{J} \exp\left(\beta'_{m|J}x\right)}, \text{ with } m = 1, \ldots, J \quad (1)$$

Replacing $\beta_{m|J} = \varphi_{\text{m}} \tilde{\beta}$ in Eq. (1) results in the stereotype model that can be written mathematically.

$$\text{Prob}(|\text{y} = \text{m}|\text{x}) = \frac{\exp\left(\varphi_m \tilde{\beta}' x\right)}{\sum_{j=1}^{J} \exp\left(\varphi_1 \tilde{\beta}' x\right)} = \frac{\exp\left(\varphi_m \tilde{\beta}_0 + \varphi_m \tilde{\beta}_1 x_1 + \ldots + \varphi_m \tilde{\beta}_k x_k\right)}{\sum_{j=1}^{J} \exp\left(\varphi_m \tilde{\beta}_0 + \varphi_m \tilde{\beta}_1 x_1 + \ldots + \varphi_m \tilde{\beta}_k x_k\right)},$$

with $m = 1, \ldots, J$

$$(2)$$

For some parameters of Eq. (2) that are not identifiable, we consider as constraints $\varphi_m \tilde{\beta}_0 \equiv \theta_m (m = 1, \ldots, J)$, where $\phi_J = 0$; and $\varphi_m \tilde{\beta}_j \equiv -\theta_m \beta_j (m = 1, \ldots, J \text{ e } j = 1, \ldots, k)$, where $\varphi_J = 0$ e $\varphi = 1$. Thus, from Eq. (2), the stereotype model can be written as follows:

$$\text{Prob}(\text{y} = \text{m}|\text{x}) = \frac{\exp\left(\theta_m - \varphi_m \beta' x\right)}{\sum_{j=1}^{J} \exp\left(\varphi_1 \beta' x\right)}, \quad (3)$$

with $m = 1, \ldots, J$ where $\theta_J = 0$, $\varphi_J = 0$ where $\varphi = 1$.

2.3.2 Interpretation of estimated coefficients

Applying logarithm in function (3) to any two categories, we get:

$$\log\left[\frac{p(Y = q/x)}{p(Y = r/x)}\right] = \left(\theta_q - \theta_r\right) - \left(\varphi_q - \varphi_r\right)\beta' x. \quad (4)$$

Applying the exponential function to the exponential function to Eq. (4), it follows

$$\Omega_{q/r} = \frac{p(Y = q/x)}{p(Y = r/x)} = \exp\left\{\left(\theta_q - \theta_r\right) - \left(\varphi_q - \varphi_r\right)\beta' x\right\}. \quad (5)$$

Eq. (5) allows us to evaluate the odds ratio before and after we add a unit to the variable x_j, that is,

$$\frac{\Omega_{q/r}(x, x_k + 1)}{\Omega_{q/r}(x, x_k)} = \exp\left\{\left(\varphi_r - \varphi_q\right)\beta_x\right\}. \tag{6}$$

The value obtained in expression (6) can be interpreted as adding a unit to the variable x_k, the odds ratio of category $\boldsymbol{r}$ varies $\exp\left\{\left(\varphi_r - \varphi_q\right)\beta_k\right\}$, keeping all other variables constant.

2.3.3 Estimation of estimated coefficients

The parameters of the stereotype model are estimated by the maximum likelihood method, in which the estimators are obtained by the system of equations given in (7) as follows:

$$\mathrm{p_i} = \begin{cases} \mathrm{Prob}(\mathrm{y_i} = 1|\mathrm{x_i}, \varphi, \theta) & \text{if } y_i = 1 \\ \vdots & \\ \mathrm{Prob}(\mathrm{y_i} = \mathrm{m}|\mathrm{x_i}, \varphi, \theta) & \text{if } y_i = m \\ \vdots & \\ \mathrm{Prob}(\mathrm{y_i} = \mathrm{J}|\mathrm{x_i}, \varphi, \theta) & \text{if } y_i = \mathrm{J} \end{cases} \tag{7}$$

where p_i is the probability of observing any value of $\boldsymbol{y}$, and the $\mathrm{Prob}(\mathrm{y_i} = 1|\mathrm{x_i}, \varphi, \theta)$ was defined in expression (3). Assuming that the sample is independent and identically distributed, the likelihood function is given by the following expression (8):

$$\mathrm{L}(\beta, \varphi, \theta|y, x) = \prod_{i=1}^{N} p_i = \prod_{m=1}^{J}\prod_{y=m}\mathrm{Prob}(\mathrm{y} = \mathrm{m}|x, \varphi, \theta) \tag{8}$$

on what $\prod_{y=j}$ indicates the multiplications over all cases where $y = m \ (m = 1, \ldots, J)$. Applying logarithm to the likelihood function obtained in (8), we obtain the logarithm of the likelihood function given in (9) as follows:

$$\log\left(\mathrm{L}(\beta, \varphi, \theta|y, x)\right) = \sum_{m=1}^{J}\sum_{y=m}\log\left[\mathrm{Prob}(\mathrm{y} = \mathrm{m}|x, \varphi, \theta)\right]. \tag{9}$$

The parameters ϕ's and θ's of Eq. (9) are estimated by the Newton–Raphson method.

The odds ratio formed will have an upward trend, as the weights can be produced by sorting. Thus, the effect of covariates on the first odds ratio is smaller than the effect on the second, and so on.

These weights can be done a priori, being estimated by a pilot study or by a set of properly chosen values.

In the case of this work, the number of disabilities that a person may have can vary from 0 to 4, and there may be five response options.

In order to assess the goodness of fit for ordinal models, it can be done using tests such as Pearson's or deviation. These tests involve creating a contingency table in which the rows consist of all possible configurations of the model's covariates and the columns are the ordinal response categories [8]. The expected counts (E_{lj}) from this table are expressed by $E_{lj} = \sum_{l=1}^{N_L} \hat{p}_{ij}$, on where N_L is the total number of individuals classified in the row l and $\hat{p}_{ij}$ represents the probability of an individual in line l having the answer j calculated from the adopted model.

Pearson's test to assess the adequacy of fit compares these expected counts with those observed by the formula:

$$\chi^2 = \sum_{l=1}^{L} \sum_{j=1}^{k} \frac{\left(O_{lj} - E_{lj}\right)^2}{E_{lj}} \tag{10}$$

The deviance stat also compares observed (O_{lj}) and expected counts, but using the formula:

$$D^2 = 2\sum_{l=1}^{L} \sum_{j=1}^{k} O_{lj} \log \frac{O_{lj}}{E_{lj}} \tag{11}$$

The tests to assess the goodness of fit of the model are given by approximations of statistics (10) and (11) for chi-square distribution with $(L-1)(k-1)p$ degrees of freedom, where L and k are as defined earlier and p is the number of model covariates. Significant differences lead to the conclusion that the model does not fit the data studied.

As an alternative, we will use the Wald test which is given by:

$$W = (\hat{p} - \hat{p}_0)' \hat{V}_p^{-1} (\hat{p} - \hat{p}_0) \tag{12}$$

on where $\hat{V}_p$ is the consistent estimator of the variance-covariance matrix of the estimator $\hat{p}$ of the proportion vector $\hat{p}$. An estimator $\hat{V}_p$ can be obtained by linearization method.

2.3.4 Significance test for the model

The Wald test for the parameters considered individually can be obtained by comparing the estimate of maximum likelihood of a given coefficient $\left(\hat{\beta}_j\right)$ with the estimate of its standard error (based on the asymptotic distribution of the maximum likelihood estimators). Thus, the null hypothesis and the alternative hypothesis of the test are respectively:

$$H_0 : \hat{\beta}_j = \beta_j^* \quad \text{vs} \quad H_1 : \hat{\beta}_j \neq \beta_j^* \qquad (\text{j} = 2, \ldots, \text{k}), \tag{13}$$

the respective statistic under the null hypothesis:

$$T = \frac{\hat{\beta}_j - \beta_j^*}{\sqrt{\text{var}\left(\hat{\beta}_j\right)}} \sim \text{N}(0, 1) \tag{14}$$

By rejecting H_0, for a significance α, we conclude that the estimated parameter is statistically different from β_j^*. Generally, use $\beta_j^* = 0$ which, under these conditions, we conclude that the parameter is relevant to explain the behavior of the dependent variable.

2.3.5 Selection of variables

Selecting variables means choosing a subset that retains the most important predictor variables in such a way that we seek to avoid problems such as multicollinearity and that this subset fits as well as the complete model and contains the most important predictor variables.

Among different procedures that can be used to select variables, we highlight forward stepwise and backward stepwise. Forward stepwise starts with the constant β_0 and sequentially adds the predictor X_i most correlated with Y to the model so that it improves the fit according to the evaluation of the F statistic and the introduction of variables when it fails to produce an F statistic greater than the 90th or 95th percentile of the distribution, $F_{1,\, N-k-2}$, where N is the sample size and k is the number of variables.

On the other hand, the backward stepwise selection strategy starts with the model with all independent variables, and sequentially, excludes variables using the F statistic to choose the predictors to be eliminated. The predictor that has the smallest F statistic is eliminated, and the process stops when each predictor eliminated from the model has an F value greater than the 90th or 95th percentile of the distribution, $F_{1,\, N-k-2}$. For this work, forward backward and the Wald statistic were chosen.

In ordinal logistic regression, the TRV (likelihood ratio test) ensures the significance of the fit. Thus, at each stage of the process, the most important variable, in statistical terms, is one that produces the greatest change in the logarithm of the likelihood in relation to the model without the variable [9].

After estimating the parameters, the next step is to verify if the covariates used for modeling are statistically significant for the modeled event, for example, condition of an individual becoming a disability person.

To test the significance of the coefficient of a covariate, it is sufficient to compare the observed values of the response variable with the predicted values obtained by the models with and without the variable of interest [10].

The comparison between observed and predicted values is made using the likelihood ratio test, which is widely applicable by the maximum likelihood estimation.

For test $H_0 : \theta \in \Theta_0$ versus $H_a : \theta \in \Theta_0^c$, we calculated the statistics [11]:

$$\lambda(x) = \frac{\sup_{\theta_0} L(\theta/x)}{\sup_{\theta} L(\theta/x)}. \text{For } n \to \infty, \; -2\ln\lambda(x) \to \chi^2_v. \tag{15}$$

where ν is obtained through the difference between the number of parameters existing in the tested model and the number of parameters existing in the saturated model [12].

To verify the quality of the adjusted model, it is sufficient to compare the observed and predicted values for the response variable (in this case, one of the different deficiencies already mentioned).

When choosing a particular model, it means that we must include as many independent variables as possible to improve the forecast; simultaneously, we want to include a smaller number of variables for reasons of cost and simplicity [10].

According to Draper and Smith [13], to select the best model is to reconcile two objectives (incorporating a certain number of variables that can improve the predictability of the model, at the same time, discarding variables that are not significant as a way of simplifying the model to reduce costs). This selection involves a dose of subjectivity, and the result may be different if the procedure is used for selection changes.

2.3.6 Model selection

Selecting a model means, after the formulation and adjustment of different plausible models, to select the model that ¨best¨ fits the data of a certain experiment according to a certain criterion adopted [14].

In statistics, there is a vast literature relevant to the selection of models [15–17]. An alternative for model selection is the use of methods based on the likelihood function that provides several statistical measures that help in the comparison between different models. The most common of these measures are as follows: Akaike Information Criterion (AIC) proposed by Paulino et al. [18] and Sakamoto et al. [19] with penalty given discounting the value of twice the difference between the number of parameters between the two models; Bayesian Information Criterion (BIC) discussed by Paulino et al. [18] and having as a penalty the value of double the number of parameters between the two models multiplied by the Naperian logarithm of the sample size; and, finally, Deviation Information Criterion (DIC) also discussed by Paulino et al. [18] and the penalty is given by the sum of the difference value between the number of parameters between the two models.

In this text, for each of the AIC, BIC, and DIC criteria, the model with the lowest value for each one of them is chosen.

2.4 Epidemiology

According to the International Epidemiology Association (IEA), epidemiology is defined as the study of the different factors involved in the spread and propagation of diseases, frequency, their mode of distribution, their evolution, and the placement of the necessary means for their prevention in human communities.

According to Suser [20], epidemiology is essentially a population science, which is based on the social sciences for the understanding of social structure and dynamics, on mathematics for statistical, probability, inference, and estimation notions, and, on the biological sciences, the knowledge of the environment organic substrate where the observed manifestations will find individual expression.

A single and precise definition of epidemiology as a scientific field ends up not being possible due to the increasing complexity and scope of its current practice:

Science that studies the health-disease process in society, analyzing population distribution and determining factors of risk, diseases, injuries, and events associated with health, proposing specific measures for the prevention, control, or eradication of diseases, damages, or health and protection problems, promotion or recovery of individual and collective health, producing information and knowledge to support decision-making in the planning, administration, and evaluation of health systems, programs, services, and actions [21].

Epidemiology is a basic discipline of public health aimed at understanding the health-disease process within populations, an aspect that differentiates it from clinical practice, which aims to study this same process, but in individual terms and that studies the different factors that intervene in the spread and propagation of diseases, their frequency, their mode of distribution, their evolution, and the placement of the necessary means for their prevention.

In scientific terms, epidemiology is based on causal reasoning; as a public health discipline, focusing on the development of a sequence of actions aimed at protecting and promoting the health of the community.

Epidemiology is also an important tool for policy development in the health sector. Its application in this case must be taken into account the available knowledge, adapting it to local realities.

Among the possibilities of applications of epidemiology, we highlight: the analysis of the health situation; identify profiles and risk factors; carry out epidemiological assessment of services; study and understand the causality of health problems; describe the clinical spectrum of diseases and their natural history; assess the performance of health services in responding to the problems and needs of populations; test the efficacy, effectiveness, and impact of intervention strategies, as well as the quality, access, and availability of health services to control, prevent, and treat health problems in the community; identify risk factors for a disease and groups of individuals who are at greater risk of being affected by a particular disease; define modes of transmission; identify and explain patterns of geographic distribution of diseases; establish methods and strategies to control health problems; establish preventive measures; assist in the planning and development of health services; and, finally, establish criteria for health surveillance.

In the discussion about disabilities, epidemiological views on social points of view, accessibility, assistive technology, among others, were used in these researches, and, physicians, from the perspective of prevention, treatment, and control.

2.5 Disability risk

According to the WHO:

- The prevalence of disabled people is high;

- The number of disabled people increases due to the aging of the population and the global improvement in chronic health conditions associated with disability such as diabetes, cardiovascular disease, and mental illness;

- Diverse experiences in which disability resulting from the interaction between health conditions, personal, and environmental factors vary widely; and finally,

- Factors such as prevalence, purchasing power, working conditions, and education are considered risks for people to become disabled. Causes like these that can aggravate this situation in vulnerable populations.

Given this scenario, reasons have emerged that justify the need to assess the well-being or disabled people life quality, we propose the creation of the risk index for disabled people, composed of the weighting of the responses of the different variables obtained from the microdata of the IBGE Census and selected as significant after applying backward stepwise methodology in an ordinal logistic regression adjustment of the stereotype type for each disability studied. This methodology gradually emerged from simpler techniques to more complex techniques such as multivariate as factor analysis.

2.6 Epidemiological risk

In the area of health, several studies on risk are located in the epidemiological area. Briefly, epidemiological risk can be summarized as the probability of the occurrence of a health-related event, estimated from the occurrence of an event that occurred in the recent past. In this way, this risk can be computed by quantifying of times the event occurred divided by the potential number of events that could have happened. In this way, the risk of becoming a disability person in a given population or group of people is the amount of disabilities persons that occurred in the previous period by the number of people existing in that period, since any person or all can potentially become a disabled person.

The definition of the epidemiological risk concept and the method incorporated by the medical area end up defining lifestyles producing meanings that guide behaviors; thus, a form of individual surveillance is articulated in a pulverized, internalized, and less visible way, translated into self-control [22].

In this work, we are considering the risk of a given person becoming a disability person, including a set of health and social factors.

3. Results and discussions

For this work, we used ordinal logistic regression analysis for each of the following response variables:

- Disabilities, which represent the number of disabilities that each person has and can assume a value between 0 and 4 disabilities;
- Disability to see, hear, and move considering the categories: 0, *"for those who cannot at all,"* 1, *"for those who can, but with great difficulty,"* 2, *"for those who can, but with a little difficulty,"* and, 3, *"for those who do not have a problem"*;
- Intellectual disability, considering the categories *"have"* or *"have not,"* and finally;
- For statistical analysis, the following programs were used SPSS, Statistica, R, and Excel.7

For this study, the variables were divided into blocks such as: identification of respondents, education, family, and work. For each of these blocks, the models were adjusted considering the variables considered significant were applied:

a. Selection of variables using the backward stepwise procedure, excluding variables that are not significant by the Wald test at each step;

b. Repeat step a) until there are no more variables to be deleted;

c. For each of these adjustments, calculate AIC, BIC, and DIC model selection criteria;

d. Select the best model among the different final models for each of the different deficiencies and number of deficiencies for the criteria: AIC, BIC, and DIC, and finally;

e. Calculate for each individual the risk of being a disability person for different degrees of severity, disability, and number of disabilities.

Figures 1–8 present in item (a) the risk graphs of being a person with one (represented by p_1 in blue dots), two (represented by p_2 in red dots), three (represented by p_3 in green dots), four disabilities (represented by p_4 in purple dots), and at least one disability (represented by p_t in black dots) and in item b) of being a visually disabled person for each different degrees of severity: "*total blind*" (represented by p_1 in blue dots); "*low vision*" (represented by p_2 in red dots); "*lighter visual*" (represented by p_3 in green dots); and, finally "*visually disability person*" (represented by *pt* in purple dots) for the variables: region in **Figure 1**, sex in **Figure 2**, age in **Figure 3**, race in **Figure 4**, education in **Figure 5**, main job in **Figure 6**, income categorized in **Figure 7**, and number of children in **Figure 8**.

In **Figure 1**, the following regions were considered: 1 – "north," 2 – "northeast," 3 – "southeast," 4 – "south," and 5 – "central west."

Starting from the graphs in **Figure 1** for the region, we see that the highest incidence risks in item a) of disability and in item b) of visual disability are found in the northeast region for all different degrees of disability and all different severity degree. In contrast, the lowest incidence rates in a) number of disabilities are found in the Midwest region and b) the lowest incidence of risk of visual disability is found in the South region.

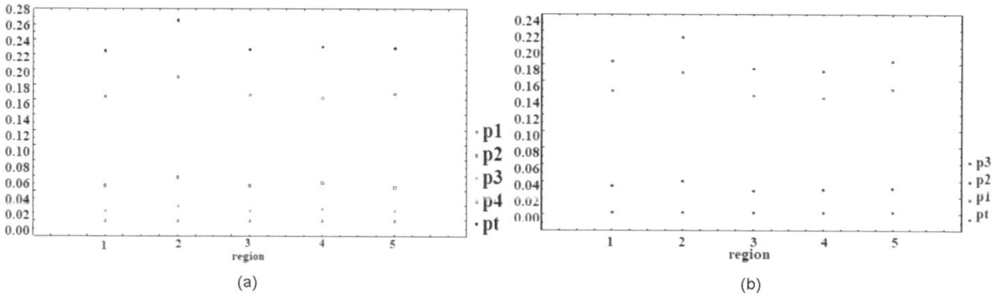

Figure 1.
Graphs of probability of occurrence: (a) of a certain number of disabilities and (b) of visual disability according to their degrees of severity for variable region.

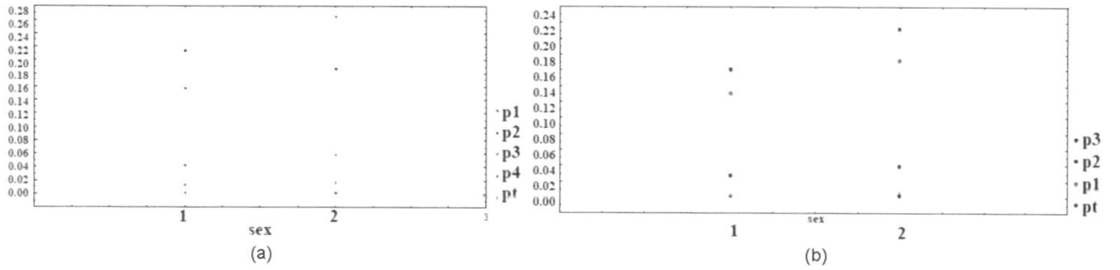

Figure 2.
Graphs of probability of occurrence: (a) of a certain number of disabilities and (b) of visual disability according to their degrees of severity for variable sex.

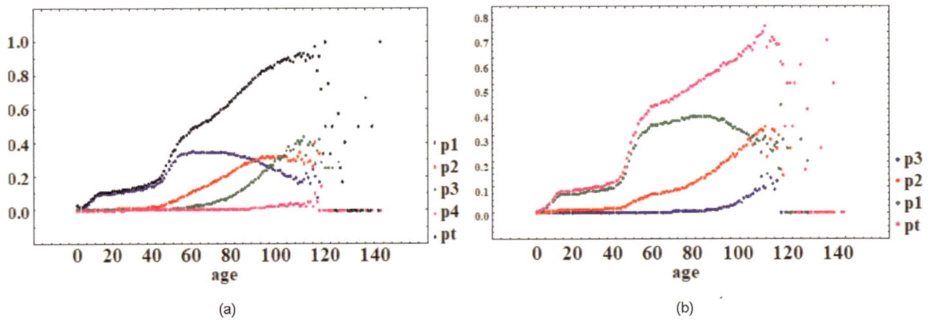

Figure 3.
Graphs of probability of occurrence (a) of a certain number of disabilities and (b) of visual disability according to their degrees of severity for age variable.

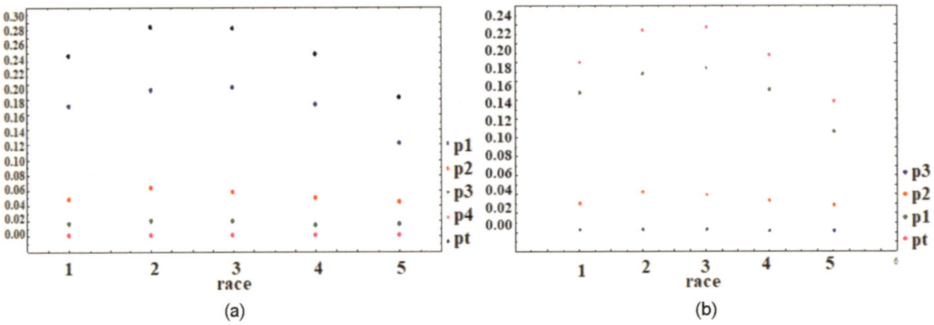

Figure 4.
Graphs of probability of occurrence (a) of a certain number of disabilities and (b) of visual disability according to their severity degrees for race variable.

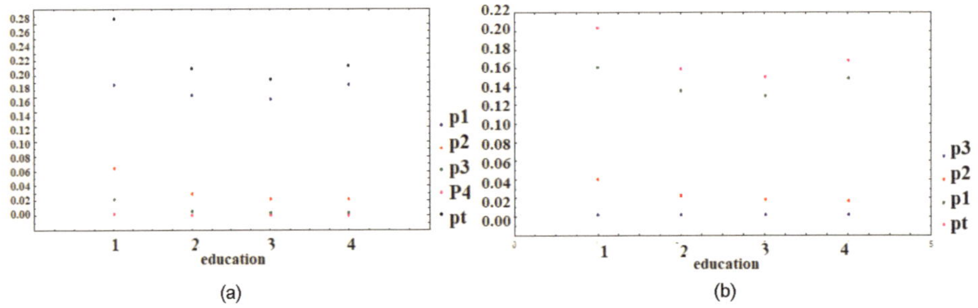

Figure 5.
Graphs of probability of occurrence (a) of a certain number of disabilities and (b) of visual disability according to their severity degrees for education.

Figure 2 shows (a) the risks of being a disabled person, and (b) the risk of incidence of visually disabled person considering genders 1 – male and 2 – female.

From the graphs in **Figure 2**, it can be seen that in all cases, the highest risk of incidence of: (a) disability and (b) visual disability is higher for females.

On the other hand, **Figure 3** presents the risks of incidence of: (a) disability and (b) visual disability as a function of age.

In **Figure 3**, it is possible to notice that the risks of disability in (a) and visual disability in (b) increase as the age of the people interviewed increases.

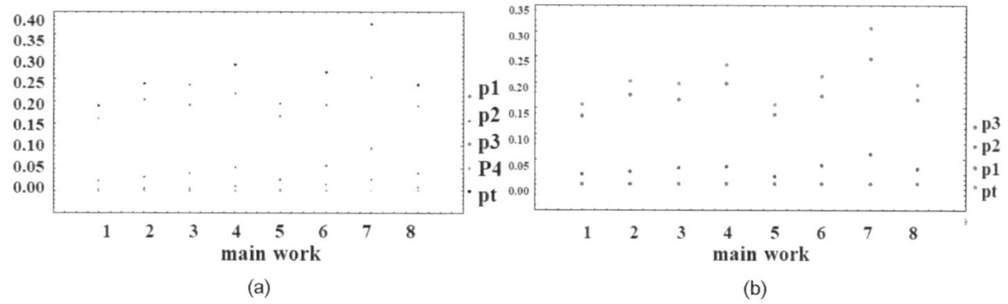

Figure 6.
Graphs of probability of occurrence (a) of a certain number of disabilities and (b) of visual disability according to their severity degree for main work.

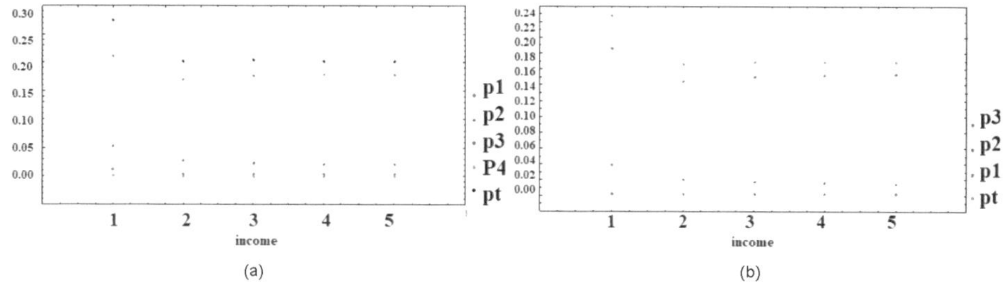

Figure 7.
Graphs of probability of occurrence (a) of a certain number of disabilities and (b) of visual disability according to their degrees of severity for income.

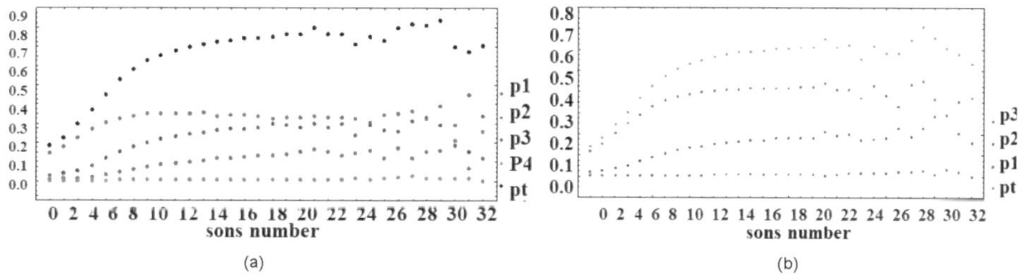

Figure 8.
Graphs of probability of occurrence (a) of a certain number of disabilities and (b) of visual disability according to their degrees of severity for number of children.

It is also noted in **Figure 3** that, from a certain age, starting at 80 years old, the points begin to be randomized, and this type of occurrence is believed to be due to a smaller number of people in these older age groups.

Foe the races in **Figure 4**, the races were defined as: 1 – White, 2 – Black, 3 – Yellow, 4 – Brown, and 5 – Indigenous.

As for the results of **Figure 4**, we note that the highest probability of occurrence of disability and visual disability is found in the Yellow race and lower in the Indigenous race.

Next, for **Figure 5**, we considered for education: 1 – "between no education and incomplete elementary," 2 – "between complete elementary and incomplete high school," 3 – "between complete high school and incomplete higher education," and, finally, 4 – "complete higher or more."

Continuing, examining **Figure 5**, we found that the highest occurrence of new cases of risk of disability and risk of visual disability is found in 1, "among no schooling and incomplete elementary school," while the lowest incidence of these risks is found in 3, "between high school complete and incomplete elementary higher education" in all situations.

For the main job in **Figure 6**, we consider the following levels: 1 – "employees with a formal contract," 2 – "military and statutory civil servants," 3 – "employees without a formal contract," 4 – "own account," 5 – "employers," 6 – "unpaid," 7 – "workers in production for their own consumption," and, finally, 8 – "total."

Observing the graphs in **Figure 6** for the type of main job, we see that the highest risk of incidence of disability and visual impairment are found in 6, "workers in production for own consumption" and the lowest risk of incidence in both cases was found in 2, "employees with a formal contract."

Continuing in **Figure 7** with income, we adopted as criterion: 1 – "between 0 and 1 minimum wage," 2 –"between 1 and 3 minimum wages," 3 – "between 3 and 7 minimum wages," 4 – "between 7 and 15 minimum wages," and, finally, 5 – "15 minimum wages or more."

From the results obtained in the graphs in **Figure 7**, we can see that the highest risk of incidence of disability and visual disability was found in 1, "between 0 and 1 minimum wage," and it is noted that this risk decreases as income increases of the person interviewed.

Finally, in **Figure 8**, a scatter plot was made for the risk of incidence of disability and visual disability as a function of the number of children.

As for **Figure 8**, it is possible to verify that the risk of disability and visual impairment increases as the number of children increases.

This result may reflect situations such as: a greater number of children can mean a greater number of accidents and less parental attention to each child in social and economic terms.

Tables 1–5 shows results for the analyses: stereotype ordinal logistic regression; selection criteria for AIC, BIC, and DIC models and for point and interval estimates of the parameters considering as response variable for the adjustments having as a response variable the deficiencies: number of disabilities (**Table 1**), visual (**Table 2**), hearing (**Table 3**), physical (**Table 4**), and intellectual (**Table 5**) marked in bold, as well as the explanatory variables included in the final model for each of the adjustments for significant variables according to the backward stepwise method.

For variable number of disabilities, we obtain the following predictor variables as significant as an adjustment for each different block:

Identification: domicile, categorized age, birthplace, nationality, and region; *Education*: reading and writing, day care, other graduation, and education; *Family*: union nature, marital status, and number of children; *Work*: income, secondary work, main work, travel, and return time; and finally; Combined model (**Table 1** – made up of all predictor variables considered significant in each of the blocks): region, place of birth, reading and writing, day care, employment status, education, union nature, marital status, number of children, income, return, and main job. For model selection, we get −7232 for AIC, −8791,418 for BIC, and − 6917,953 for DIC.

As for visual disability, the following variables were selected: Identification: region, domicile, sex, birthplace, and nationality; Education: reading and writing, day care, other graduation, and education; Family: union nature, marital status, and number of children; Work: income, time, condition, situation, and secondary work, and finally; Combined model (**Table 2**) initialized with all explanatory variables that were

Variables		Estimatives	Standard errors	Wald	df	p-value	Confidence interval 95%	
							Lower limit	Upper limit
Disabilities	0	−.210	.075	7.786	1	.005	−.358	−.063
	1	1.922	.075	650.417	1	.000	1.774	2.070
	2	3.938	.077	2636.890	1	.000	3.787	4.088
	3	7.034	.104	4562.783	1	.000	6.830	7.238
Region	1	.250	.013	365.872	1	.000	.225	.276
	2	.295	.011	714.216	1	.000	.273	.317
	3	−.071	.010	51.179	1	.000	−.090	−.051
	4	−.181	.011	281.285	1	.000	−.202	−.160
	5	0			0			
Naturalness	1	−.060	.006	97.127	1	.000	−.072	−.048
	2	.076	.014	31.279	1	.000	.049	.103
	3	0			0			
Read and write	1	−.428	.015	869.893	1	.000	−.456	−.399
	2	0			0			
Childcare	1	−.022	.023	.953	1	.329	−.066	.022
	2	−.114	.024	21.574	1	.000	−.162	−.066
	3	−.012	.019	.412	1	.521	−.050	.025
	4	0			0			
Occupation condition	1	.086	.059	2.130	1	.144	−.029	.201
	2	−.205	.059	12.091	1	.001	−.320	−.089
	3	−.405	.059	47.319	1	.000	−.520	−.289
	4	−.486	.059	67.149	1	.000	−.602	−.370
	5	0[a]			0			
Instruction level	1	.037	.014	7.143	1	.008	.010	.063
	2	−.060	.014	17.007	1	.000	−.088	−.031
	3	−.006	.017	.118	1	.731	−.039	.028
	4	0			0			
Union nature	1	.297	.014	473.400	1	.000	.270	.324
	2	.480	.024	411.506	1	.000	.434	.527
	3	.561	.016	1209.135	1	.000	.529	.592
	4	.819	.023	1244.424	1	.000	.773	.864
	5	0			0			
Marital status	1	−1.055	.015	5009.257	1	.000	−1.084	−1.026
	2	−.909	.013	5024.643	1	.000	−.934	−.884
	3	−.509	.013	1621.905	1	.000	−.534	−.485
	4	0			0			

Variables		Estimatives	Standard errors	Wald	df	p-value	Confidence interval 95%	
							Lower limit	Upper limit
Income	1	.304	.032	89.934	1	.000	.241	.367
	2	.171	.032	29.101	1	.000	.109	.233
	3	.170	.032	28.047	1	.000	.107	.233
	4	.133	.035	14.378	1	.000	.064	.202
	5	0			0			
Return	1	−.221	.017	174.562	1	.000	−.254	−.188
	2	0			0			
Main job	1	−.209	.023	79.698	1	.000	−.255	−.163
	2	−.460	.135	11.602	1	.001	−.724	−.195
	3	.066	.025	7.006	1	.008	.017	.114
	4	−.131	.023	31.478	1	.000	−.176	−.085
	5	−.066	.024	7.620	1	.006	−.113	−.019
	6	−.428	.032	180.577	1	.000	−.491	−.366
	7	0			0			

Table 1.
Point and interval estimates of the parameters of the logistic model considering the number of deficiencies (deficiencies) as the response variable.

considered significant for each of the different blocks and were selected: region, birthplace, read and write, day care, education, union nature, number of children, return, condition, and situation. For model selection, we get −2549,708 for AIC, −3291,833 for BIC, and finally −2399,707 for DIC.

Next, for hearing disability, the following variables were selected for each of the different blocks: Identification: region, domicile, sex, race, and birthplace; *Education*: reading and writing, day care, other graduation, and education; *Family*: union nature, marital status, and number of children; *Work*: income, time, condition, situation, main work, and secondary work; and finally, *Joint model* (**Table 3**): region, birthplace, reading and writing, education, marital status, number of children, condition, and situation. For model selection, we get −2921.348 for AIC, −3331.401 for BIC, and −2865.348 for DIC.

For physical disability, the following variables were selected: *Identification*: region, age, and birthplace; *Education*: reading and writing, day care, other graduation, and education; *Family*: union nature, marital status, and number of children; *Work*: income, return, time, condition, situation, main work, and secondary work; and finally, *Joint model* (**Table 4**): region, birthplace, reading and writing, day care, education, marital status, number of children, return, time, condition, situation, and main job. For model selection, we get AIC = −1258.613, BIC = −2119.480, and DIC = −1084.013.

Finally, in the case of **Table 5**, the following variables were selected as significant: gender, age, birthplace, knowing how to read and write, and education. Totally, there are five variables.

Variables		Estimatives	Standard errors	Wald	df	p-value	Confidence interval 95%	
							Lower limit	Upper limit
Visual disability	1	−5.190	.072	5147.165	1	.000	−5.332	−5.048
	2	−2.012	.066	935.571	1	.000	−2.141	−1.883
	3	.177	.066	7.310	1	.007	.049	.306
	4	10.966	.140	6174.537	1	.000	10.692	11.239
Region	1	−.272	.013	421.476	1	.000	−.298	−.246
	2	−.262	.011	544.896	1	.000	−.284	−.240
	3	.141	.010	193.114	1	.000	.121	.161
	4	.275	.011	609.290	1	.000	.253	.297
	5	0			0			
Naturalness	1	.051	.006	67.199	1	.000	.039	.064
	2	−.077	.014	30.191	1	.000	−.105	−.050
	3	0			0			
Read and write	1	.369	.014	710.297	1	.000	.342	.396
	2	0			0			
Childcare	1	−.041	.022	3.940	1	.049	−.084	.002
	2	.043	.024	3.098	1	.078	−.005	.091
	3	−.018	.019	.931	1	.335	−.054	.018
	4	0			0			
Instruction level	1	−.062	.060	1.064	1	.302	−.181	.056
	2	.226	.060	14.015	1	.000	.108	.345
	3	.425	.060	49.529	1	.000	.307	.544
	4	.460	.061	57.577	1	.000	.341	.579
	5	0			0			
Union nature	1	−.223	.007	1108.625	1	.000	−.236	−.210
	2	−.135	.008	260.276	1	.000	−.151	−.118
	3	−.067	.016	17.005	1	.000	−.099	−.035
	4	0			0			
Children	1	1.101	.015	5656.802	1	.000	1.072	1.130
	2	.922	.012	5599.102	1	.000	.898	.946
	3	.498	.012	1696.917	1	.000	.474	.522
	4	0			0			
Return	1	.213	.016	166.427	1	.000	.180	.245
	2	0			0			
Condition	1	0			0			
Situation	1	0			0			

Table 2.
Point and interval estimates of the logistic model parameters considering visual disability as the response variable.

Variables		Estimatives	Standard errors	Wald	df	p-value	Confidence interval 95%	
							Lower limit	Upper limit
Hearing disability	1	−6.251	.081	5885.079	1	.000	−6.410	−6.091
	2	−4.350	.079	3058.665	1	.000	−4.504	−4.196
	3	−2.495	.078	1017.060	1	.000	−2.648	−2.342
	4	12.767	.288	1962.330	1	.000	12.202	13.332
Region	1	−.098	.018	29.749	1	.000	−.133	−.063
	2	−.299	.015	401.518	1	.000	−.329	−.270
	3	−.015	.014	1.204	1	.273	−.043	.012
	4	.005	.015	.131	1	.718	−.024	.035
	5	0			0			
Naturalness	1	.039	.008	22.219	1	.000	.023	.055
	2	−.110	.018	38.663	1	.000	−.145	−.075
	3	0			0			
Read and write	1	.449	.012	1302.286	1	.000	.424	.473
	2	0			0			
Instruction level	1	−.445	.075	35.178	1	.000	−.592	−.298
	2	−.119	.075	2.475	1	.116	−.266	.029
	3	.123	.075	2.688	1	.101	−.024	.271
	4	.292	.076	14.760	1	.000	.143	.441
	5	0			0			
Marital status	1	−.122	.009	177.545	1	.000	−.139	−.104
	2	−.395	.021	352.262	1	.000	−.436	−.354
	3	−.468	.016	824.993	1	.000	−.500	−.436
	4	−.816	.014	3433.926	1	.000	−.843	−.789
	5	0			0			
Children	1	.826	.016	2645.864	1	.000	.795	.858
	2	.709	.013	2870.222	1	.000	.683	.735
	3	.432	.012	1207.655	1	.000	.407	.456
	4	0			0			
Condition	1	.042	.014	9.356	1	.002	.015	.068
	2	0			0			
Situation	1	0			0			
	2	0			0			

Table 3.
Point and interval estimates of the parameters of the logistic model considering hearing disability as the response variable.

Variables		Estimatives	Standard errors	Wald	df	p-value	Confidence Interval 95%	
							Lower limit	Upper limit
Walk disability	1	−5.591	.125	1987.299	1	.000	−5.837	−5.345
	2	−2.726	.120	512.061	1	.000	−2.962	−2.490
	3	−1.146	.120	90.832	1	.000	−1.382	−.911
	4	13.027	.234	3110.980	1	.000	12.569	13.485
Region	1	−.182	.022	71.172	1	.000	−.224	−.139
	2	−.370	.018	436.802	1	.000	−.404	−.335
	3	−.086	.016	28.375	1	.000	−.118	−.055
	4	−.047	.018	7.112	1	.008	−.082	−.013
	5	0			0			
Naturalness	1	.012	.010	1.576	1	.209	−.007	.031
	2	−.157	.020	60.058	1	.000	−.197	−.117
	3	0			0			
Read and write	1	.577	.017	1171.179	1	.000	.544	.610
	2	0			0			
Childcare	1	.333	.029	133.621	1	.000	.277	.390
	2	.586	.039	220.779	1	.000	.509	.664
	3	−.025	.022	1.311	1	.252	−.068	.018
	4	0			0			
Instruction level	1	−.569	.109	27.157	1	.000	−.783	−.355
	2	−.104	.109	.908	1	.341	−.319	.110
	3	.267	0.109	5.963	1	.015	.053	.482
	4	.538	0.11	23.881	1	.000	.322	.754
	5	0			0			
Marital status	1	−.125	.010	142.810	1	.000	−.146	−.105
	2	−.530	.022	585.604	1	.000	−.572	−.487
	3	−.621	.017	1326.137	1	.000	−.654	−.588
	4	−.933	.016	3244.635	1	.000	−.965	−.901
	5	0			0			
Children	1	1.009	.020	2554.328	1	.000	.970	1.049
	2	.794	.016	2471.085	1	.000	.763	.825
	3	.382	.015	639.566	1	.000	.352	411
	4	0			0			
Return	1	0			0			

Variables		Estimatives	Standard errors	Wald	df	p-value	Confidence Interval 95%	
							Lower limit	Upper limit
Time	1	.691	.031	506.529	1	.000	.631	.751
	2	.673	.029	524.780	1	.000	.615	.73
	3	.508	.030	283.211	1	.000	.449	.568
	4	.284	.032	80.361	1	.000	.222	.346
	5	0			0			
Condition	1	0			0			
Situation	1	0			0			
Main job	1	.542	.033	266.774	1	.000	.477	.607
	2	.497	.241	4.229	1	.040	.023	.970
	3	−.010	.036	.076	1	.783	−.080	.060
	4	.415	.033	158.503	1	.000	.351	.480
	5	.216	.034	40.930	1	.000	.150	.283
	6	.623	.053	139.555	1	.000	.520	.727
	7	0			0			

Table 4.
Point and interval estimates of the parameters of the logistic model considering physical disability as response variable.

In intellectual ability, the following variables were selected: *Identification*: region, sex, age, race, and birthplace; *Education*: reading and writing, day care, other graduation, and education; *Family*: union nature, marital status, and number of children; *Work*: income, time, return, condition, situation, and secondary work; and finally, *Joint model*: gender, age, birthplace, reading and writing, and education. For model selection, we get AIC = −14,548. BIC = −14,711, and DIC = −14,515.

Making a comparative study between the models given in **Tables 1–5**, we noticed that the model that included a smaller number of variables was the logistic model adjusted for intellectual disability, while the model that required the largest number of independent variables was for the number of deficiencies.

The adjustment by stereotype ordinal logistic regression was compared with binary logistic regression [1] and multinomial logistic regression [23], and visual, hearing, physical, intellectual, and multiple disabilities were considered.

It was found that, for all the different disabilities, the one that had the highest number of independent variables considered significant was for the regression methodology, binary logistic followed by the stereotype ordinal logistic regression methodology, and this can be motivated by the following facts:

To enable the use of dummy variables, the response variable had to be transformed to determine whether or not it has a disability, which increased the sensitivity of the analysis, making differences more easily detected.

The stereotype logistic regression methodology performed better in relation to the multinomial logistic regression methodology, as it took into account that the response categories were ordinal, contrary to what happened when the multinomial logistic

Variables		Estimatives	Standard errors	Wald	df	p-value	Confidence interval 95%	
							Lower limit	Upper limit
Intellectual disability	1	−3.795	.087	1923.902	1	.000	−3.964	−3.625
	2	10.498	.096	11945.597	1	.000	10.310	10.686
Sex	1	−.103	.006	284.656	1	.000	−.115	−.091
	2	0			0			
Age	1	.664	.013	2719.203	1	.000	.639	.689
	2	.073	.008	84.007	1	.000	.057	.089
	3	0			0			
Naturalness	1	−.139	.007	454.576	1	.000	−.152	−.126
	2	−.251	.015	274.087	1	.000	−.281	−.221
	3	0			0			
Read and write	1	1.486	.007	46829.311	1	.000	1.473	1.500
	2	0			0			
Instruction level	1	−.943	.086	120.203	1	.000	−1.112	−.775
	2	−.303	.087	12.254	1	.000	−.473	−.133
	3	.116	.087	1.802	1	.179	−.054	.286
	4	.362	.089	16.647	1	.000	.188	.535
	5	0			0			

Table 5.
Point and interval estimates of the parameters of the logistic model considering as the answer variable intellectual disability.

regression model was applied, and this probably caused that the multinomial logistic regression methodology has little sensitivity and presents a smaller number of selected variables in the composition of its models [24].

Among the advantages of using multinomial logistic regression, we can mention the fact of not making assumptions about the probabilistic behavior of the independent variables, possibility of testing the significance of a large number of independent variables, and, finally, possibility of direct estimation of the probability of an observation belonging to a certain class [25, 26].

4. Conclusions

The adjusted model with the lowest number of explanatory variables was the intellectual one with 5, while the one that needed the highest number was disability with 13 variables.

In this work, using the ordinal stereotype ordinal logistic model, it was possible to improve the quality of the fit when compared to the fit of the binary logistic model proposed in Oliveira [1]. When using the ordinal response, the disability risk was incorporated for different severity degrees and disabilities number.

The different deficiencies are not homogeneous, as for different predictor variables.

The incidence risks of being a disability person and being a visual disability person are probably greater in situations such as residing in the northeast region, female gender, aged over 80 years, Yellow race, incomplete elementary education, working in production for their own consumption, and high number of children.

The lower incidence risks are observed in situations such as residing in the southern region, male gender, aged 15 years or less, Indigenous race, schooling between complete high school and incomplete higher education, and worker with a formal contract and without children.

Next, for **Figures 1–8**, we proceed to establish possible justifications and suggestions for work or research that may or may not accept the considered hypotheses.

- **Figure 1**. These results may be occurring due to the low effective investment in terms of health and infrastructure, smaller in the northeast and north regions, and larger in regions like the southeast and south.

To evaluate this hypothesis, an alternative is to carry out a survey of the effective volume spent on health, accessibility, and infrastructure that favor disabled people between the different regions, counting the number of people who were effectively benefited and make a comparative assessment between the different regions;

- **Figure 2**: These are most likely results that reflect women's greater exposure to domestic accidents and the double shift of modern women who work outside the home and take care of the home.

To better assess this point, the proposal can be a comparative study by sampling between the times of work at home and outside the home between men and women;

- **Figure 3**: These results show that with the aging of the population over the years, with greater life expectancy and more subject to diseases of advanced age and a greater incidence of becoming disabled people.

In this case, it is possible to suggest studies that simultaneously prove the increase in life expectancy of the population and the emergence of diseases that occur at more advanced ages. This point can be easily confirmed by the data from the 2010 IBGE Census Sample;

- **Figure 4**: These results show cultural and dietary conditions of Eastern and Indigenous peoples.

For a better understanding of this result, we suggest a research study on the life habits of Yellow and Indigenous people races, considering their possibilities of becoming disabled people;

- **Figure 5**: It is believed that a low education can mean less knowledge of information, low purchasing power, and greater dependence on government aid.

In order to prove it, research can be carried out that can establish relationships between level of education and income;

- **Figure 6**: Most likely, the different types of professions reflect the education obtained by different workers, since being military or statutory depends on passing a public tender that requires better preparation and study, while I work for my own consumption or without pay, in general, it is made up of people who work in the countryside, are unemployed and have lower purchasing power.

In order to better evaluate this possibility, the proposal is to carry out research that can establish the average remuneration for different professions by disability, sex, education, and other demographic variables;

- **Figure 7**: The higher incidence of risk can be justified as it tends to be higher when the population's purchasing power or income is lower.

In this case, we suggest a study in which a survey is carried out on disabled people and without disabilities and then, visual disabled people and without visual disability, and that we make a comparison between different income levels; and finally;

- **Figure 8**: This result may reflect situations such as a greater number of children can mean an increase in the number of accidents and less attention paid to each child by the parents in social and economic terms.

In this case, to show this result, it suggests the establishment of a survey that can compare life quality among families with different numbers of children and evaluate their respective risk.

For **Figures 1–8**, the results were similar for the amount of disabilities and visual disability.

The conclusions of this work verify, in addition, the importance of other studies, researches, and analyses, because, when talking about risk, there are several methods to assess this risk, whether using regression coefficients, whether using regression analysis, factor scores, weighting of the disability risk considering the weighting of the risk for each of the different explanatory variables. For example, disability risk is known to increase as age increases, so does the number of children, and so on. Among various alternatives for future work, we can mention the following ones:

1. Beta regression model, factor analysis, structural equation modeling, and the BART algorithm as a way to improve the goodness of fit and its reliability in determining the deficiency index.

2. Repeat the analysis including variables related to housing conditions and possession of other assets.

3. Among several questions that need to be answered are questions about how disabled people live and what situation they find themselves in when buying them from people without disabilities.

4. In situations like this, a risk index with good reliability and adjustment quality is interesting to facilitate the monitoring of this situation, in the same way as with

the Human Development Index (HDI), although this is a more general index, still does not take into account the issue of disabled people.

5. Evaluate the accessibility of the surroundings of the houses of disabled people, considering the locations in a georeferenced way, evaluating the conditions of the infrastructure proposing a geostatistical model.

6. The difficulty in estimating the risk index is to obtain a method that is efficient and reliable and that manages to reduce its discrepancy. Due to this problem, it ends up becoming of interest on the part of researchers, making the use of several methods to be able to estimate this risk considered and evaluated in this study.

7. The advantage of having an index that can be compared is that it can be used as a parameter to see if its value has increased or decreased, in such a way that the higher this index should reflect the greater need for intervention by public authorities to reduce the existing barriers in terms of access to different human rights and accessibility around the homes of disabled people.

8. Propose improvements in the census questionnaire, for example, if a respondent answered that he is a disability person, also ask at what age it occurred, because, according to the existing literature [3], it is known that the older the age people become disabled people, the greater the difficulties for that person to adapt.

9. In statistical terms, improve national statistics on disability, using an efficient and low-cost approach to obtain more comprehensive data and add disability questions, cross-reference between different datasets, collect longitudinal data, add disability issues to allow monitoring, improve data comparability, develop adequate tools, fill gaps between investigations and, finally, strengthen and support the different investigations considering the creation of instruments that can measure and monitor life quality and the well-being of these people on a continuous and periodic basis.

10. Also include issues related to health conditions, housing, work, education, accessibility, and leisure.

11. Repeat the analysis by region, state, and municipalities.

12. It is hoped that results such as this research can contribute to the action of public managers with better support in meeting the needs of disabled people.

Acknowledgements

The author thanks IBGE for accessing the microdata of the selected households to compose the sample and Professor Julia Maria Pavan Soler for indicating the topic.

Author details

Paulo Tadeu Meira e Silva de Oliveira
University of São Paulo, São Paulo, Brazil

*Address all correspondence to: poliver@usp.br

References

[1] Oliveira PTMS. Pessoas com deficiência: análise dos resultados do Censo 2010 e a sua evolução. In: 58 RBRAS/15 SEAGRO, in the period from July 22 to 26 2013. Brazil: Campina Grande – PB; 2013

[2] Silva OM. A epopeia ignorada. São Paulo-SP, Brazil: CEDAS; 1987

[3] Garcia VG. Disabled People and the Labor Market. Brazil: Economic Institut – UNICAMP; 2010

[4] Figueira E. Caminhando em silêncio. São Paulo: Giz editorial e Livraria Ltda; 2008

[5] Agresti A. An Introduction to Categorical Data Analysis. Florida, USA: Wiley & Sons; 2019

[6] Anderson JA. Regression and ordered categorical variables. Journal of Royal Statistics Society. 1984;**16**:1-30

[7] Paulino CD, Singer JM. Análise de dados categorizados. Blucher: Editora Edgard; 2006

[8] Abreu MNS. Uso de modelos de regressão logística ordinal em epidemiologia: um exemplo usando a qualidade de vida. Belo: Public Heralth College; 2007

[9] Hastie T, Tibshirani P, Friedmann J. The Elements of Learning: Data Mining, Inference and Population. Canada: Springer; 2009

[10] Oliveira PTMS. Application of the Genetic Algorithm in the Mapping of Epistatic Genes in Controlled Crosses. São Paulo, Brazil: IME-USP; 2008

[11] Casella G, Berker PL. Statistical Inference. Brooks, California: EUA; 1990

[12] Oliveira PTMS. Estimation and Hypothesis Testing in Comparative Calibration. São Paulo: IME-USP; 2001

[13] Draper NR, Smith H. Applied Regression Analysis. New York: Jonh Wiley; 1998

[14] Camarinha-Filho JA. Mixed Linear Models: Estimates of Variance and Covariance Matrices and Model Selection. Brazil: ESDALQ-USP; 2008

[15] Broman K. Identifying Quantitative Trait Locos in Experimental Cross. Berkeley: University of California; 1997

[16] Burnham KP, Anderson DR. Model Selection and Multimodel Inference. New York: Springer; 2002

[17] Burnham KP, Anderson DR. Model Selection and Inference. New York: Springer; 1998

[18] Paulino CD, Turkman AA, Murteira BJF. Estatística Bayesiana. Portugal: Fundação Calouste Gulbenkian; 2003

[19] Sakamoto Y, Ishguru M, Kitamura G. Akaike Information Criterion Statistics. Japon: KTK, Scientific Publisher; 1986

[20] Suser M. Epidemiology, Health & Society – Selected Papers. New York: Oxford University press; 1987

[21] Almeida Filho N, Rouquayrol MZ. Introdução a epidemiologia moderna. Rio de Janeiro: Guanabara Koogan; 2006

[22] Luiz OC, Cohn A. Sociedade de risco e risco epidemiológico. Rio de Janeiro: Cadernos Saúde Pública; 2006

[23] Oliveira PTMS. Disabilities people: some analysis of the 2010 Census results

and its evolution. In: 58 RBRAS/ 15 SEAGRO, 2013, from July 22 to 26. Campina Grande-PB; 2014

[24] Abreu MNS, Siqueira AL, Caiaffa WT. Ordinal logistic regression in epidemiological studies. Rev. Saúde Pública. 2009;**43**:1

[25] Oliveira PTMS. Pessoas com deficiência: questão de risco sob aplicação de regressão logística politômica e sob visão epidemiológica. In: XIV School Regression Models, 2015, from March 2 to 5, Convention Center, UNICAMP, Campinas-SP, Program and Abstracts. Brazilian Statistical Association; 2015

[26] Oliveira PTMS. Disabled People in Brazil: Risk Question. 2018. Available from: https://www.preprints.org/manuscript/201802.0171/v1

Chapter 2

The Basics of Structural Equations in Medicine and Health Sciences

Ramón Reyes-Carreto, Flaviano Godinez-Jaimes and María Guzmán-Martínez

Abstract

Structural Equation Models (SEM) are very useful and, with a wide range of practical applications in many fields of science, in medicine and health sciences, have increased interest in their usefulness. This chapter is divided into three sections. The first includes concepts, notation, and theoretical aspects of SEM, such as path diagrams, measurement model, confirmatory factor analysis, structural regression, and identification model. In addition, it includes some simple examples applied to health sciences. The second section deals with the estimation and evaluation of the model. On the first topic, the methods of Maximum Likelihood (ML), Generalized Least Squares, Unweighted Least Squares, and ML with robust standard errors are addressed, as well as alternative methods to the problem of violations of the multivariate normality assumption. On the second topic, some goodness of fit statistics of the estimated model are defined, such as the chi-square statistic, Root Mean Square Error of Approximation, Tucker-Lewis Index, Comparative Fit Index, Standardized Root Mean Square Residual, and Goodness of Fit Index. The last section deals with SEM example and its implementation using the lavaan library of R software.

Keywords: causal effects, path diagram, measurement model, confirmatory factor analysis, structural regression

1. Introduction

SEM is a multivariate method whose use has grown exponentially in medicine and health sciences. The SEM is a statistical method considered as a causal model that includes, among other techniques, the Linear Regression Model (LRM), Factor Analysis (FA), Confirmatory Factor Analysis (CFA), and Path Analysis. This statistical model can help the researcher to test or confirm theoretical models or hypotheses and validate causal relations between variables, which can be latent and observed, or only between observed variables.

When a researcher is interested in investigating the causal relationships between a grouping of variables that define a factor or latent variable, he is interested in proving or confirming (or discontinuing) that his hypothetical model is appropriate for the data analyzed.

As a result, the researcher has the following options: a) when the hypothetical model is confirmed by the analyzed data, he can include new elements to the original model and then analyze that new structure; b) when the hypothetical model is not appropriate for the analyzed data, the original model can be modified or a new model can be tested.

Pearl cited by Kline [1] defines SEM as a causal method that considers as input (a) a set of qualitative causal hypotheses based on theory or the results of empirical studies represented by a set of equations, (b) a set of questions about the causal relationship between factors or latent variables of interest. Many SEM applications focus on non-experimental or observational designs and data from quasi-experimental or experimental designs.

2. Variables and path diagram in health and medicine

2.1 Causality

SEM models assume probabilistic causality. This allows changes in the results to occur with a probability between 0 and 1.0. The estimation of effects using the data is founded on probability distribution assumptions; thus, causality is understood as a functional relationship between two quantitative variables, effects change a probability distribution. Causality assumptions for a researcher in Medicine and Health are done through a synthesis of logic, theory, and prior knowledge, in this way the causal relationship between observed and latent variables is conceptually hypothesized with expert clinical judgment [2].

The SEM includes observed or manifest variables, latent variables, errors or disturbances, and parameters. There are two main ways to communicate and understand the equations that the SEM represents: through simultaneous equations or by a path diagram. A path diagram is a visualization of the conceptual model, and a conceptual model is an idea of the relationship under study. Behind the ideas of causal inference are Bayesian networks and causal graphs; for example, a causal directed graph can include, common causes, whether measured or unmeasured variables.

2.2 Observed, latent variables, disturbances, and effects

Observed variables are measured and recorded in the data (e.g. sex, age, height, weight, systolic blood pressure, diastolic blood pressure, body mass index). In a path diagram, these variables are represented by rectangles or a box. A standardized variable is a variable that has a mean zero and a variance one. Latent variables or latent constructs are variables that are not directly measured (e.g. depression, metabolic syndrome, obesity, and anxiety). In a path diagram, they are described by circles or ovals. Observed or latent variables can be exogenous or endogenous. Exogenous variables are variables that are not influenced (not caused) by others variables in a model. This variable is the cause or effect of one or more variables in the model. Endogenous variables are those variables that are influenced by other variables. An endogenous variable can affect another variable of the same type.

Disturbances are the unspecified causes of the effect variable. Each endogenous variable is assigned a disturbance, and this is considered as a latent variable.

Effects can be direct, indirect, and totals. These effects can be represented by directed lines. The direct effect (→) is the causal effect of an independent variable on another called dependent, that is, the direct influence of one variable on another. Any variable can be strictly independent (exogenous) or a dependent variable or endogenous.

Indirect effect is a causal effect of an independent variable on a dependent through the pathway of a third variable. This effect is synonymous with the mediation effect. The total effect is the sum of all possible effects of one independent variable on another dependent. All the effects are estimated by various techniques from the sample data.

2.3 Path diagram

It is a graphical description of an SEM that includes a measurement model and a structural model, where measured or observed variables are represented by rectangles, latent variables by circles, and curved lines represent unanalyzed associations. The covariances or correlations between exogenous variables are described by a curved line with two arrowheads. The variance is represented by two-headed curved arrows on the same variable observed or latent. Here, the latent variables are treated as continuous in what we shall refer to as conventional SEM (or what is sometimes called first-generation SEM). Hypothesized causal effects or direct effects, on endogenous variables, are represented by a line with a single arrowhead.

Kline [1] on parameters of SEM, when means are not included, suggests defining parameters in words that are parallel to three symbols utilized in Reticular Action Model (RAM) symbolis a direct effect, on endogenous variables, is represented by a line with a single arrowhead; double-headed curved arrows that go out and re-enter the same variable, represent the variance of an exogenous variable; and the double-headed curved arrows entering one variable and leaving another variable to represent the covariance.

In medicine and health sciences, it is common to assess a latent variable by several observed variables, for example, obesity can be indirectly measured by the observed variables percentage of fat (FAT), body mass index (BMI), and abdominal circumference (AC) (**Figure 1**).

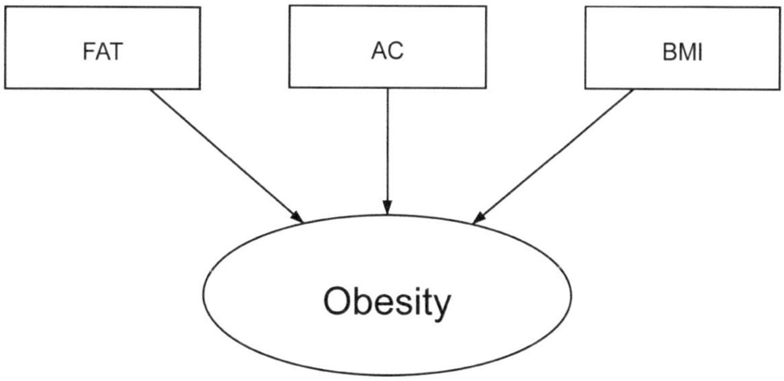

Figure 1.
A path diagram representing the latent variable obesity measured by three observed variables: Percentage of FAT (FAT), body mass index (BMI), and abdominal circumference (AC).

3. Measurement and structural models

In medicine and health sciences, it is common to use one of the four types of SEM that exist in the literature. Next, each one is briefly described.

Path analysis models: This method of SEM only includes observed variables, similar that multiple regression models (MRM), but it has the advantage that a variable can be a dependent variable and an independent variable at the same time, in addition, there can be several dependent variables, and the indirect and direct effects can be measured (**Figure 2**). In **Figure 2** (below), the Socioeconomic Status (SES) and Disease, both exogenous variables, represent direct effects on the endogenous variable obesity.

Confirmatory Factor Analysis models (CFA): The CFA, like the measurement model, analyzes the relation among latent and observed variables, emphasizing that the theoretical factorial structure predetermined by the researcher is confirmed by the data; that is, it must be predetermined to which factor the observed variables will be loaded and the CFA will be useful to confirm or not the default structure.

Structural Regression Model: This method of SEM is a regression model between latent variables. The idea consists on to combine the techniques of CFA and MRM, further include the measurement errors.

The causal relationships between latent variables are represented by the directional arrows according to the hypothetical model. Typically, model fit indices are examined first, followed by hypothesis tests. The latent growth curve model is a statistical technique of longitudinal analysis that estimates or explains the growth over a period of time.

In this chapter, we will only address the Structural Regression Model.

3.1 Measurement model

This part of the path diagram is necessary to analyze all the items or observed variables that are "loaded" in the latent variable, their variances, and errors, as well as the relation between the observed variables.

The measurement model quantifies linkages among the latent variables and observed variables that characterize the hypothetical model.

The latent variables are representations of the concepts of interest. Previously the concept is selected, Bollen [4] recommends for the measurement process: (1) Determine its meaning, (2) Represent it with latent variables, (3) Form measures, and (4) Establish the relation among latent variables and measures variables.

The measurement model analyzes the relation between the measure and latent variables. The latent variable is the representation of a concept. This relation can be described or represented by an equation or in a path diagram (**Figure 3**).

The CFA is a method for evaluating a measurement model. Klein [1] mentioning Bollen suggests applying some rules to ensure the identification of the measurement model re specifying it as a CFA. When it comes to a CFA, a factor must have at least three observed variables, when there are two or more factors or latent variables each factor must have at least two observed variables.

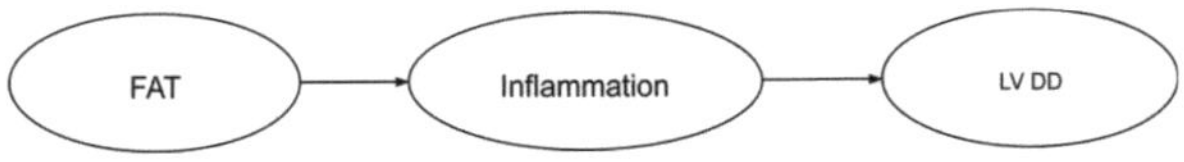

Figure 2.
The path diagram above represents the indirect effect between FAT and LV diastolic dysfunction, and the path diagram below shows the direct effects of socioeconomic status and obesity, and between disease and obesity [3].

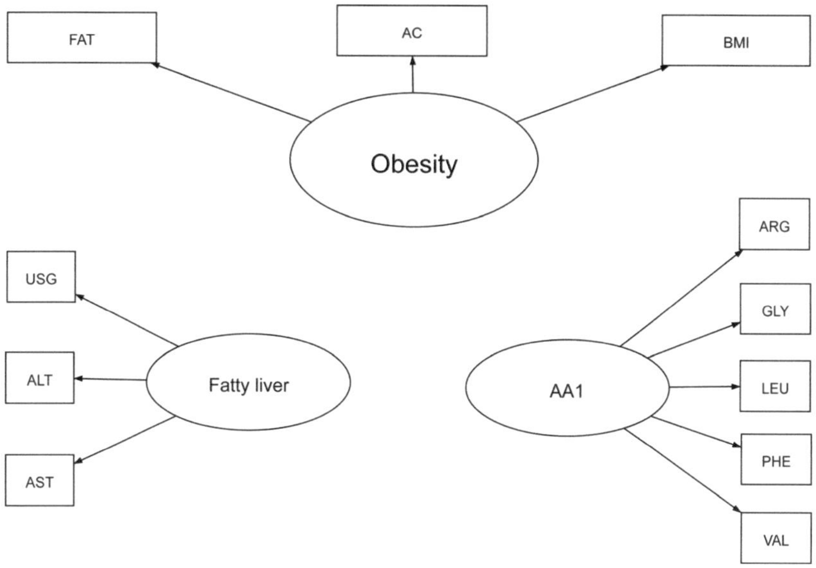

Figure 3.
A path diagram of the CFA model on Matsuda index with 11 observed variables: Percentage of FAT (FAT), body mass index (BMI), abdominal circumference (AC), arginine (ARG), glycine (GLY), leucine (LEU), phenylalanine (PHE), valine (VAL), liver ultrasound (USG), alanine aminotransferase (ALT), aspartate aminotransferase (AST); and 3 latent variables: Amino acids (AA1), fatty liver, and obesity [5].

3.2 Structural regression model

The path diagram of structural regression (SR) includes the set of latent variables and their relationships. Unlike the measurement model (CFA) where all the factors or latent variables are exogenous and can be assumed to covary or have a dependency, the causal effects between latent variables are described only in the SR. Causal inference in latent variable modeling is more laborious than measurement model analysis. In SR models the effects between latent variables can also be direct or indirect. Similarly, the structural component can also be recursive or non-recursive. A recursive SR is a model in which causation is directed in one single direction, while a non-recursive structural model has causality going in both directions on some variables.

3.3 Identification of SR model

Identification of the SR model is analogous to the identification of the measurement model. However, before validating the SR, the measurement model needs to be identified (i.e., valid) and then evaluate the fully SEM model. The only valid identification of the CFA does not guarantee the identification of the SR.

Therefore, the analysis of a fully SEM must include the variances and covariances between the factors or latent variables A fully SR model is identified by [4]: (1) In the first, the researcher must analyze the measurement model as a CFA, that is, ignore in the analysis the relations among the latent variables of the SR model. After reformulating the model, discover if the model is identified. If identification is obtained, apply it to the second step; (2) in the second step, you must analyze the equation or equations that contain the relation among the latent variables of the SR model must be analyzed and

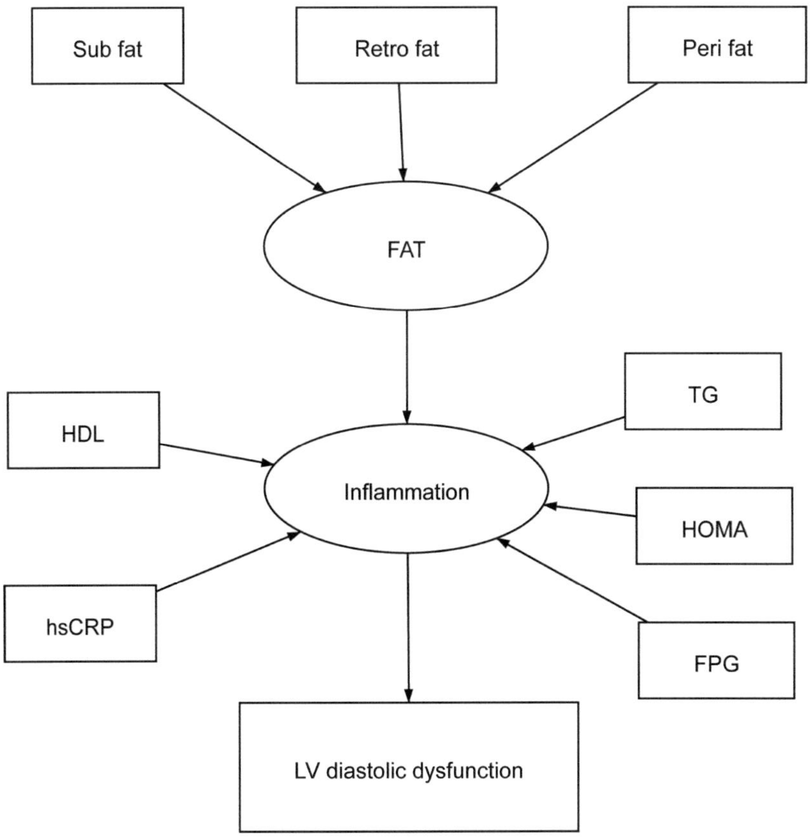

Figure 4.
SEM to analyze relationships between adiposity, inflammatory responses, LV diastolic dysfunction. Fasting plasma glucose (FPG); high-density lipoprotein (HDL); homeostasis model of insulin resistance (HOMA); high sensitivity C-reactive protein (hsCRP); peritoneum fat area (Peri fat); retroperitoneum fat area (retro fat); subcutaneous fat area (sub fat); triglyceride (TG). The latent variable FAT directly influences the inflammation variable and indirectly on the observed variable LV diastolic [6].

then determine if the SR model is identified, assuming that the latent variables are observed variables. If in step 1 it is proved that the measurement parameters are identified and in step 2 that the parameters of the SR are also identified, both conditions are sufficient to fully identify the SR model. **Figure 4** shows a path diagram of a complete SEM, which includes 9 observed variables and two latent variables. The objective is to analyze the relationship among central obesity (FAT), systemic inflammation (Inflammation), and left ventricular diastolic dysfunction (LV diastolic). This figure does not show the variances or the disturbances or errors.

4. Equations and model estimation

4.1 The equations

The basic goal of SEM is to generalize the CFA to assess relationships between latent variables [7]. A classic form of SEM representation is the LISREL model which involves a measurement model and a structural model. The measurement model defines the relationship between the latent variables and their indicators or observed variables, and the structural model defines the relationship between the latent variables. In this section, we will address the linear SEM model and the nonlinear case.

The measurement equations are:

$$\mathrm{x} = \Lambda_x \xi + \delta \quad (1)$$

$$\mathrm{y} = \Lambda_y \eta + \varepsilon \quad (2)$$

In Eq. (1), $\boldsymbol{x}$ is the vector of observed exogenous variables, $\boldsymbol{\xi}$ is the vector of exogenous latent variables, $\boldsymbol{\delta}$ is the vector of errors and $\Lambda_{\boldsymbol{x}}$ the matrix of coefficients that relates $\boldsymbol{x}$ to $\boldsymbol{\xi}$. In Eq. (2), $\boldsymbol{y}$ is vector of observed variables referred to as endogenous, $\boldsymbol{\eta}$ is the vector of latent variables also endogenous; $\boldsymbol{\varepsilon}$ is the vector of errors for the endogenous variables, and $\Lambda_{\boldsymbol{y}}$ the matrix of coefficients relating $\boldsymbol{y}$ to $\boldsymbol{\eta}$. In addition, connected with the two previous equations we have the covariance matrices: Θ_δ and Θ_ε are the matrix of covariances among errors $\boldsymbol{\delta}$ and ε, respectively.

In summary, the object of the measurement model is to analyze the relation of the latent variables in ξ and η with the observed variables in x and y, respectively. One problem in formulating these equations is to specify the factorial loading matrix Λ, based on a priori information on the observed and latent variables considered in the study.

The structural equation for linear SEMs is:

$$\eta = \Gamma\xi + \zeta \quad (3)$$

The structural equation for nonlinear SEMs is:

$$\eta = B\eta + \Gamma\xi + \zeta \quad (4)$$

where $\boldsymbol{\eta}$ is the vector of endogenous variables, $\boldsymbol{\xi}$ is the vector of exogenous variables, and $\boldsymbol{\zeta}$ explain the latent errors of endogenous variables; and $\boldsymbol{B}$ is the matrix of coefficients that explain the relation among endogenous latent variables, Γ explain the linear effects of exogenous variables on endogenous, and $\boldsymbol{\zeta}$ include of errors of endogenous variables. Related to Eq. (4) we have the following matrices: Φ and Ψ are the covariance matrix of latent exogenous variables and the matrix of covariances among errors of endogenous variables, respectively.

4.2 Assumptions and limitations

Normality: The most important assumption in SEM is the multivariate normal distribution (MVN), particularly when the maximum likelihood (ML) method is used to estimate the model parameters. When discrete variables have used the assumption of normality is violated. The violation or omission of the assumption of the MVN of the observed variables leads to a high value of χ^2_M/df_M and to an affectation of the significance of the test. In this scenario, it is suggested to apply other methods such as Generalized Least Squared (GLS).

When the complexity of the SEM increases, the sample size must also increase, and when the data depart from the normal distribution it is essential to increase the number of observations [1]. The non-normality assumption can be detected by univariate tests, multivariate tests, and skewness and kurtosis statistics. The skewness and kurtosis can be measured, separately or together in the same variable. In the context of SEM, the kurtosis is more problematic than skewness in terms of the effects on inference. If the absolute value of the skewness exceeds 2 and kurtosis exceeds 4, then the distribution is non-normal [8].

No correlation between errors: The errors are assumed to be independent, that is, there is no correlation between the errors $\boldsymbol{\delta}, \boldsymbol{\varepsilon}$ and $\boldsymbol{\zeta}$.

Multicollinearity: It is assumed that there is no strong relationship among the independent variables.

Linearity: It is assumed that exists linear relation among the variables.

Outliers: The presence of outliers in the data affects the significant results of the model.

Sample size: Generally, the number of observations in the sample affects the results of the fit indices in SEM. [9] suggest a minimum sample size of 150; [10] suggest at least 10 times the number of parameters in the model: [11] recommends should be at least 200, and Hair et al. mentioned by Thakkar [12] provides an interesting list. However, if the number of observations is small, it is reasonable and recommendable to use the Bayesian approach of SEM.

Limitations: Prior to analysis, and since the SEM model is a statistical method of confirmation, the researcher must establish a hypothetical model, analyze the model based on the sample and the latent, and observed variables. Additionally, one must know how many parameters you need to estimate, adding variances, covariances, and path coefficients. Of course, one must know all the relationships that he/she intends to specify in the model.

4.3 Estimation

Let $\Sigma = \Sigma(\boldsymbol{\theta})$ be the covariance matrix of the model, where Σ is the population matrix corresponding to the observed variables, $\boldsymbol{\theta}$ is a vector of (unknown) parameters, and $\Sigma(\theta)$ is a matrix as a function of $\boldsymbol{\theta}$, which is estimated by minimizing the discrepancy among a sample covariance matrix S and $\Sigma(\theta)$. The estimation methods minimize different discrepancy functions F between S and $\Sigma(\boldsymbol{\theta})$, so that

$$F = \min(S, \Sigma) \tag{5}$$

where the matrix $\Sigma(\boldsymbol{\theta})$ is given by

$$\begin{aligned}\Sigma(\theta) &= \begin{bmatrix} E(yy^T) & E(yx^T) \\ E(xy^T) & E(xx^T) \end{bmatrix} = \begin{bmatrix} \Sigma_{yy}(\theta) & \Sigma_{yx}(\theta) \\ \Sigma_{xy}(\theta) & \Sigma_{xx}(\theta) \end{bmatrix} \\ &= \begin{bmatrix} \Lambda_y C(\Gamma\Phi\Gamma^T + \Psi)C^T {\Lambda_y}^T + \Theta_\varepsilon & \Lambda_y C\Gamma\Lambda{\Lambda_x}^T \\ \Lambda_x \Phi \Gamma^T \mathbf{C}^T {\Lambda_y}^T & \Lambda_x \Phi {\Lambda_x}^T + \Theta_\delta \end{bmatrix}\end{aligned} \tag{6}$$

Note that this matrix does not depend on observed or latent variables but on the matrices of unknown parameters $\Theta_\delta, \Theta_\varepsilon, \Phi, \Psi, \Lambda_x, \Lambda_y, \Gamma$ and $\boldsymbol{B}$, where $\boldsymbol{C} = (\boldsymbol{I} - \boldsymbol{B})^{-1}$.

ML estimation: In this method, function (7) is the logarithm of the likelihood, the loglikelihood. Maximization is accomplished by deriving the loglikelihood with respect to the parameters, equating each derivative to zero, and solving the equations system. This procedure requires that the endogenous variables have an MVN distribution, **S** Wishart distribution, that the observations are distributed independently and identically, and that the matrices Σ and **S** are positive definite.

$$F_{\mathrm{ML}} = log\,|\Sigma(\theta)| + tr\left(S\Sigma(\theta)^{-1}\right) - log\,|S| - tr\left(SS^{-1}\right) \tag{7}$$

where $\log()$ is the natural logarithm function, $|\cdot|$ is the determinant and $tr()$ is the trace function.

The ML estimator has among others the following advantages: is asymptotically consistent, unbiased, efficient, and the model fit statistic T_{ML} is asymptotically distributed as χ^2 with $df = \frac{p(p+1)}{2} - t$, where t is the number of model parameters estimated.

Two other estimation methods that consider endogenous variables with MVN distributions are generalized least squares (GLS) and unweighted least squares (ULS), which are described below.

GLS estimator: This method is a member of a family known as fully weighted least squares (WLS) estimation, which is suggested to be applied when the data is considered severely non-normal; in addition, it has the property of being asymptotically MVN distributed. The function to minimize is given by

$$F_{\mathrm{GLS}} = \frac{1}{2}\mathrm{tr}\left\{\left[I - \Sigma(\theta)S^{-1}\right]^2\right\} \tag{8}$$

ULS estimator: The method consists of minimizing the sum of squares of the differences among the sample covariance matrix and the predicted covariance matrix. This method can generate unbiased estimates but is not as good as the ML method [13]. The function to minimize is

$$F_{\mathrm{ULS}} = \frac{1}{2}\mathrm{tr}\left\{S - \Sigma(\theta)^2\right\} \tag{9}$$

In general, the ML estimator is preferred over both GLS and ULS, especially when the number of observations is large.

GLS estimator requires well-specified models but allows small sample sizes to do an acceptable job in terms of theoretical and empirical fit. WLS estimator also requires well-specified models, but in contrast to GLS and ML, it also requires large sample sizes to perform well [14]. In general, the ML estimator is preferred over both GLS and ULS, especially when the number of observations is large.

4.4 Model assessment

The SEM tests a hypothetical theoretical model about the relation among latent and observed variables, the goal of model evaluation consists in test the causal relationships of a model. There are several criteria for evaluating the fit of an SEM, so it is difficult to adopt a single specific model fit criterion. The researcher generally uses three criteria to assess the statistical significance and the substantive significance of a hypothesized model [15]:

1. The non-significance of the chi-square test indicates that the proposed model fits the data.

2. The statistical significance of individual parameter estimates is applied as a t or z value, and are compared to a t or normal distributions.

3. The magnitude and direction are positive or negative of the parameter estimates.

Kline [1], Schumacker and Lomax [15], Thakkar [12] and Douglas [2] provided indices and criteria for evaluating the fit of the model. This chapter only presents some indices: A statistical test and four basic fit statistics criteria.

a. Chi-square χ^2_M with its degrees of freedom df_M and p value.

This statistic is based on a function of the fitting function F_{ML} (7) and is given by

$$\chi^2_M = (n-1)F_{\mathrm{ML}} \tag{10}$$

where n is sample size and χ^2_M has a central chi-square distribution with degrees of freedom $df_M = p^* - t$, where $p^* = p(p+1)/2$ is the total number of variances and covariance terms, p is the number of observed variables, and t is the total number of free parameters. Among the problems that this statistic presents are that its value can be affected by the sample size, non-normality, correlation, and unique variance. To decrease the sensitivity of the χ^2_M to sample size, it is common to divide this statistic by its expected value, that is to say χ^2_M/df_M, change that reduces the value of this ratio for $df_M > 1$ compared with χ^2_M. This statistic is used to test the absolute model fit. The null hypothesis of equal fit is that there is no difference between the proposed model and the data. A large value of statistics χ^2_M with a respective small p value imply that model does not fit the data well.

b. Root Mean Square Error of Approximation (RMSEA) and its 90% confidence interval.

The RMSEA is a function of χ^2_M statistics defined by

$$RMSEA = \sqrt{\frac{\hat{\delta}_M}{\mathrm{df}_M\ (n-1)}} \tag{11}$$

where $\hat{\delta}_M = \max\left(0, \chi^2_M - df\right)$ is the estimated noncentrality parameter and χ^2_M is defined in (10).

c. The Comparative Fit Index (CFI).

Let I be the null (independence) model and its χ^2_I statistic which is approximately central chi-square distributed with degrees of freedom df_I. The CFI can be obtained using the ML estimator. This index is given by:

$$CFI = 1 - \frac{\chi^2_M - \mathrm{df}_M}{\chi^2_I - \mathrm{df}_I} \tag{12}$$

d. Goodness of Fit Index (GFI)

Model fit value	Rule of Thumb Guidelines	
Absolute fit indices	**Excellent**	**Acceptable**
Chi-square	$p \geq 0.05$	Smaller values
CFI	≥ 0.95	≥ 0.90
RMSEA	≤ 0.05	≤ 0.08
SRMR	≤ 0.05	≤ 0.08

Table 1.
Guidelines in SEM for select model fit statistics and indices [2].

GFI is the amount of variances and covariances jointly accounted for by the model. It is given by:

$$GFI = 1 - \frac{\mathrm{tr}\left(\Sigma(\theta)^{-1}S - I\right)^2}{\mathrm{tr}\left(\Sigma(\theta)^{-1}S\right)^2} \tag{13}$$

GFI varies from 0 to 1.0.

e. Standardized Root Mean Square Residual (SRMR).

SRMR is an absolute fit index that is a badness-of-fit statistic that consists of standardizing the Root Mean Square Residual (RMR). It is a measure of the mean absolute covariance residual. An SRMR = 0 means an ideal model fit, and increasingly higher values indicate a worse fit [1].

In **Table 1** a summary is given about the interpretation of the most important goodness of fit indices.

5. SEM example

5.1 Database

To illustrate the application of the packages lavaan of the R software, data from a study carried out in a Public Maternal Hospital in the state of Guerrero, Mexico, are used. The database corresponds to a cross-sectional study of pregnant women who presented to the emergency department of the Maternal Hospital with a clinical picture compatible with an obstetric emergency [16]. Two groups of patients were constituted, one group was treated from January 2009 to December 2011, which corresponds to the period before the implementation of a process called Red Code (Before RC), which is aimed at pregnant women with obstetric emergency situations; and another group of patients treated from September 2013 to December 2015, in which the Red Code (RC) procedure was implemented. The observed variables are the same for both cases, and the number of observations for the RC period is 106 and 230 for Before RC. The code and analysis presented below correspond to data from the CR period. For the Before CR case, it is a similar way. Since these are two different data sets, it is not possible to apply an analysis of variance. Therefore, to compare the results of the studied models, only the fit indices and the coefficients of factor loadings and regression are compared.

SEM is based on the variance/covariance matrix of the observed variables. However, when the observed variables present very different variances, it is suggested to use the correlation matrix. The R software is available on GNU GPL (General Public License) on the CRAN website (Comprehensive R Archive Network) https://CRAN.-R-project.org [17]. To implement SEM using the lavaan [18] package, you first need to install it using the instructions:

```
install.packages("lavaan").
library(lavaan).
```

In this data set, the opinions of the expert medical personnel assigned to the Maternal Hospital are considered to determine the following latent variables and observed variables: First Hemodynamic State (FHS) is made up of the variables observed: Temperature (Tm1), heart rate (HR1), blood pressure (BP1), respiratory rate (BF1) and the number of seizures (NC). The latent variable Second Hemodynamic State (SHS) is made up of the observed variables: Temperature (Tm2), heart rate (HR2), blood pressure (BP2), respiratory rate (BF2). Gyneco-obstetric background (OGH) is measured by the variables number of abortions (NumAb), number of cesarean sections (NumCa), weight of the pregnant woman (PW), and number of vaginal deliveries (NVD). Treatment (Treat) formed by Plasma (PLAS), platelets (PLAT), and erythrocyte concentrates (EC).

Results of the Emergency Obstetric Care (Remoc) that measure the consequences of the actions carried out in the RC process, which are the number of sequelae (NumS), the weight of the newborn (NW) in kilograms, and the weeks of gestation (GW).

5.2 Model specification

In this example, it applies the function SEM of library lavaan, which uses the correlation matrix, *Cor.RC*, and the number of observations *N.RC*. The *fit.RC* object is created, where lavaan stores the results of our SEM.

```
    ### Model especification.
Sm.RC<-'.
FHS =~ BP1 + BF1 + HR1 + Tm1 + NC.
SHS =~ HR2 + Tm2 + BP2 + BF2.
OGH =~ PW + NVD + NumAb + NumCa.
Treat =~ PLAT + PLAS + EC.
Remoc =~ NumS + NW + GW.
#### Structural model.
FHS ~ OGH.
SHS ~ FHS.
Treat ~ OGH + FHS + SHS.
Remoc ~ Treat + OGH + FHS + SHS.
'
fit.RC<-sem(Sm.RC, sample.cov= Cor.RC, sample.nobs = N.RC).
```

	Before RC	RC	Reference
Chi-square	295.5	156.0	
	p-value = 0.00	p-value = 0.216	
CFI	0.803	0.915	≥ 0.90
RMSEA	0.068 (0.057–0.079)	0.029 (0.000–0.056)	0.05–0.08
	p-value = 0.004	p-value = 0.887	
SRMR	0.078	0.087	≤ 0.08
AGFI	0.852	0.827	

Table 2.
Goodness of fit indices for the two SEMs.

5.3 Model assessment

The estimation method used in this example is the maximum likelihood method. To obtain results, it is common to use the function *summary* that provides the results of the chi-square test, the indices for the adjustment of the model (RMSEA, CFI, AGFI, among others), the estimations of the factor loads, the coefficients of regression, standard errors, Z values, and p values for each estimated coefficient. In this example, only the estimates for both periods are included, since we are interested in identifying the change or effect in each parameter estimate.

`summary(fit.RC, fit.measures= TRUE).`

It is common that before interpreting the results of the fitted model, it is necessary to verify that the fit is suitable. **Table 2** presents the results of chi-square, degrees of freedom, p-value and some fit indices to make decisions about evaluating the fit of the model for Before RC and RC case.

The chi-square results for the case of RD period are better than those of Before RD. Because the chi-square statistic is sensitive to sample size, correlation size, and non-normality, it is suggested that other adjustment indices be used. However, since there is no consensus on which goodness of fit index is the best to use, several of the indices available in the lavaan library of the R software are used here. The results of the goodness of fit indices: (a) CFI: 0.915 for RD is greater than 0.803 for Before RD, and is greater than the reference value (≥ 0.90); (b) the value of RMSEA for RD (0.029) is less than Before RD (0.068), and is even less than the reference value (0.05–0.08); and (c) the SRMR value for Before RD is less than for the RD case, both results very close to the reference value (≤ 0.08).

Finally, the values of AGFI for both periods Before RD and RD are close to the reference value of 0.90. In summary, according to the General Rules Guidelines in the SEM literature for selecting indices and model fit statistics, cited by [1, 2], these results indicate a good fit of both models, in particular, for the RD case.

5.4 Model interpretation

The interpretation for FHS is as follows: in the Before RC period, when the FHS increases by one unit, then BP1, BF1, HR1, Tm1, and NC increase by 1.0, 1.41, 1.73, 1.33, and 0.55, respectively. While for the RC period, when FHS increases by one unit, then BP1, HR1, and Tm1 increase by 1.0, 4.4, and 0.10, respectively, but BF1 and NC decrease by 1.76 and 1.98, respectively. The interpretation of the other latent variables is done in a similar way.

The observed variables that have the greatest impact or effect on each latent variable in the measurement model are: (a) In FHS: BF1 in both periods Before RC and RC (1.41 and − 1.76, respectively) and HR1 for Before RC (1.73) and for RC (4.40).

Additionally, all the factor loadings for Before RC are Significant, while for the RC period are Not Significant; (b) In SHS: All factor loadings have similar effects in both periods and also resulted in NS; (c) In OGH: the effect of NVD increased from 2.58 for the Before RC period to 30.96 for the RC period. In contrast, the effect of NumAb decreased from 0.84 for Before RC to −6.99 for period RC. However, all loads resulted in NS in both periods; (d) In Treat: The effect of the PLAS variable increased from 0.95 of the Before RC period to 1.48 of the RC period. In this latent variable, all factor loadings were significant in both periods; and (e) In Remoc: the effects of the observed variables NW and GW increased from the Before RC period to the RC period from −13.85 to 5.65 and from −18.22 to 5.14, respectively; however, all factor loadings were NS.

Although the results presented in **Table 3**, for the structural model, in both periods, are not significant, it can be said that: (a) when OGH increases one unit, then FHS increases 0.11 units in the Before RC period, but decreases by 1.27 units in the RC

Measurement model					**Structural model**				
LV	**Before RC**		**RC**		**LV**	**Before RC**		**RC**	
FHS =					FHS				
BP1	1.000		1.000		OGH	0.111	NS	−1.270	NS
BF1	1.410	***	−1.755	NS	SHS				
HR1	1.729	***	4.401	NS	FHS	1.224	***	−0.248	NS
Tm1	1.333	***	0.103	NS	Treat				
NC	0.548	***	−1.978	NS	OGH	1.194	NS	−8.185	NS
SHS =					FHS	−0.182	NS	−0.174	NS
HR2	1.000		1.000		SHS	0.354	NS	−0.251	NS
Tm2	0.491	***	0.497	NS	Remoc				
BP2	0.803	***	0.201	NS	Treat	0.010	NS	0.087	NS
BF2	0.563	***	0.650	NS	OGH	−0.042	NS	0.478	NS
OGH =					FHS	−0.062	NS	−0.054	NS
PW	1.000		1.000		SHS	0.017	NS	0.010	NS
NVD	2.579	NS	30.956	NS					
NumAb	0.838	NS	−6.993	NS					
NumCa	−0.978	NS	0.381	NS					
Treat =									
PLAT	1.000		1.000						
PLAS	0.949	***	1.483	***					
EC	0.407	***	0.531	***					
Remoc =									
NumS	1.000		1.000						

Measurement model					Structural model		
LV	**Before RC**		**RC**		**LV**	**Before RC**	**RC**
NW	−13.848	NS	5.654	NS			
GW	−18.224	NS	5.138	NS			

LV: Latent variable model, NS: Non significant.
****: P(>|Z|) < 0.05. That is, a value of statistical significance less than 0.05.*

Table 3.
Estimates of the measurement model and structural model for both models.

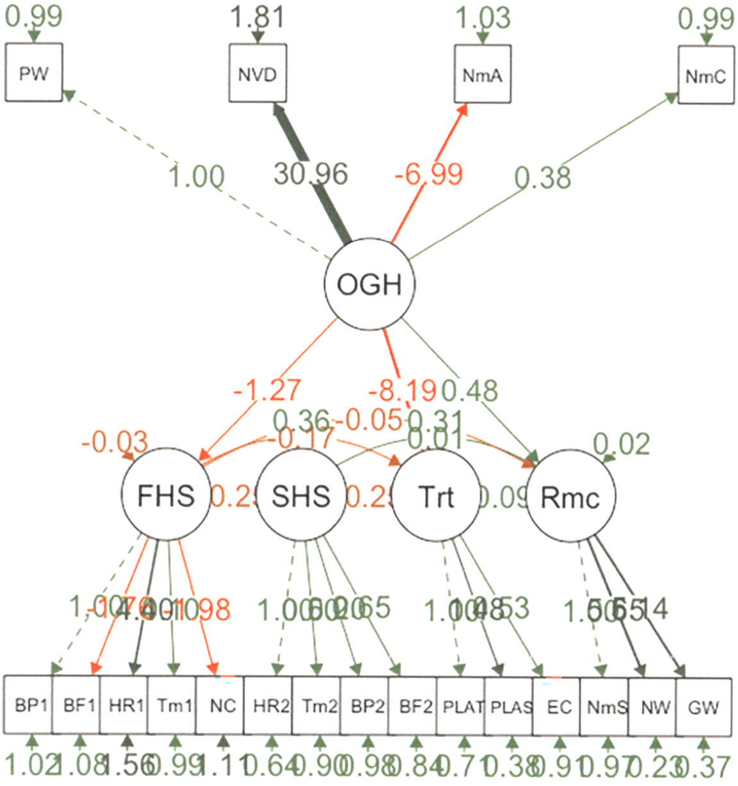

Figure 5.
Diagram path of SEM for RC period.

period; (b) When FHS increases by one unit, then SHS increases by 1.23 units in the Before RC period, but decreases by 0.25 units in the RC period. In a similar way, the other interpretations of the results of the structural model are made in both periods.

Finally, it is convenient to say that although the number of observations corresponding to the Before RC (230) is greater than the total number of observations to the RC period (106), the results of the fit indices are better for the RC case.

5.5 Results in a path diagram

It is quite common and useful to display the SEM results in a route diagram, for which the following semPlot package function can be used.

```
semPaths(fit_RD, "par", edge.label.cex = 1.2, fade = FALSE,
         style="lisrel", layout = "tree").
```

Figure 5 corresponds to the case of the RC period, it shows the final diagram of the model established in the model specification section, as well as the values of the estimates. Negative effects are shown in red and positive effects in green.

6. Conclusions

In summary, it can be concluded that there was a positive effect on the health status of patients treated with the RC process compared to patients who were not treated. The results of this study can provide information that allows the design of hospital management strategies for pregnant women with high morbidity to improve the quality of service, but in a particular way, for the Hospital de la Madre y el Nio Guerrense they can help in the care of their service. Finally, the contribution of this proposed SEM, in addition to helping to understand the management and interpretation of the model, can help to evaluate the effects of emergency obstetric care, using some observed and latent variables.

Conflict of interest

The authors declare no conflict of interest.

Abbreviations

AGFI	Adjusted Goodness of Fit Index
BMI	Body Mass Index
CFI	Comparative Fit Index
CFA	Confirmatory Factor Analysis
CRAN	Comprehensive R Archive Network
FA	Factor Analysis
GFI	Goodness of Fit Index
GLS	General Least Squares
LRM	Linear Regression Model
ML	Maximum Likelihood
MRM	Multiple Regression Models
MVN	Multivariate Normal Distribution
PA	Path Analysis
RAM	Reticular Action Model
RC	Red Code
RMSEA	Root Mean Square Error of Approximation
SEM	Structural Equation Models
SR	Structural Regression
SRMR	Standardized Root Mean Square Residual
TLI	Tucker-Lewis Index
ULS	Unweighted Least Squares
LISREL	Linear Structural Relations

Author details

Ramón Reyes-Carreto*†, Flaviano Godinez-Jaimes† and María Guzmán-Martínez†
Facultad de Matemticas, Universidad Autnoma de Guerrero, Maestra en Matemticas Aplicadas, Chilpancingo de los Bravo, Mexico

*Address all correspondence to: rcarreto@uagro.mx

† These authors contributed equally.

References

[1] Kline RB. Principles and Practice of Structural Equation Modeling. 4th ed. New York: Guilford Press; 2016

[2] Gunzler DD, Perzynski AT, Carle AC. Structural Equation Modeling for Health and Medicine. Chapman & Hall/CRC; 2021. p. 299

[3] Darbandi M, Najafi F, Pasdar Y, Mostafaei S, Rezaeian S. Factors associated with overweight and obesity in adults using structural equation model: Mediation effect of physical activity and dietary pattern. Eating and Weight Disorders-Studies on Anorexia, Bulimia and Obesity. 2020;**25**(6):1561-1571. DOI: 10.1007/s40519-019-00793-7

[4] Bollen KA. Structural Equations with Latent Variables. John Wiley & Sons; 1989

[5] Romero-Ibarguengoitia ME, Vadillo-Ortega F, Caballero AE, Ibarra-Gonzlez H-RA, Serratos-Canales MF, et al. Family history and obesity in youth, their effect on acylcarnitine/aminoacids metabolomics and non-alcoholic fatty liver disease (NAFLD). Structural equation modeling approach. PLoS One. 2018;**13**(2):1-17. DOI: 10.1371/journal.pone.0193138

[6] Wu CK, Yang CY, Lin JW, Hsieh HJ, Chiu FC, Chen JJ, et al. The relationship among central obesity, systemic inflammation, and left ventricular diastolic dysfunction as determined by structural equation modeling. Obesity. 2012;**20**(4):730-737

[7] Lee SY. Structural Equations Modeling: A Bayesian Approach. John Wiley & Sons; 2007. p. 432

[8] Kim HY. Statistical notes for clinical researchers: Assessing normal distribution using skewness and kurtosis. Restorative Dentistry and Endodontics. 2013;**38**(1):52-54

[9] Bentler PM, Chou C-P. Practical issues in structural modeling. Sociological Methods Research. 1987; **16**(1):78-117

[10] Jayaram J, Kannan V, Tan K. Influence of initiators on supply chain value creation. International Journal of Production Research. 2004;**42**(20): 4377-4399

[11] Celik HE, Yilmaz V. Lisrel 9.1 ile Yapisal Esitlik Modellemesi. Ankara: Ani Yayincilik; 2013

[12] Thakkar JJ. Structural Equation Modelling. Applications for Research and Practice (with AMOS and R). Singapore: Springer; 2020. p. 124. DOI: 10.1007/978-981-15-3793-6

[13] Kaplan D, Depaoli S. Bayesian Structural Equation Modeling, Handbook of Structural Equation Modeling. New York: The Guilford Press; 2012. pp. 650-673

[14] Olsson UH, Foss T, Troye SV, Howell RD. The performance of ML, GLS, and WLS estimation in structural equation modeling under conditions of misspecification and nonnormality. Structural Equation Modeling. 2000; 7(4):557-595

[15] Schumacker RE, Lomax RG. A Beginners Guide to Structural Equation Modeling. Routlege: Taylor & Francis; 2016

[16] Prez-Castro E, Godnez-Jaimes F, Barrera-Rodrguez E, Reyes-Carreto R, Lpez-Roque R, Vera-Leyva, V. Impact of

the red code process using structural equation models. In: Antoniano-Villalobos I, Mena, R, Mendoza M, Naranjo L, Nieto-Barajas L. (eds). Selected Contributions on Statistics and Data Science in Latin America. FNE 2018. Springer Proceedings in Mathematics Statistics. Springer, Cham; 2018. p. 111-125. DOI: 10.1007/978-3-030-31551-1_9

[17] R Core Team. R a Language and Environment for Statistical Computing. Vienna, Austria: R Foundation for Statistical Computing; 2017

[18] Rosseel Y. Lavaan: An R package for structural equation modeling. Journal of Statistical Software. 2012;**48**(2):1-36

Chapter 3

Modelling Agitation-Sedation (A-S) in ICU: An Empirical Transition and Time to Event Analysis of Poor and Good Tracking between Nurses Scores and Automated A-S Measures

Irene Hudson

Abstract

Sedation in the intensive care unit (ICU) is challenging, as both over- and under-sedation are detrimental. Optimal sedation and analgesic strategies, are a challenge in ICU and nurses play a major role in assessing a patient's agitation levels. Assessing the severity of agitation is a difficult clinical problem as variability related to drug metabolism for each patient. Multi-state models provide a framework for modelling complex event histories. Quantities of interest are mainly the transition probabilities e.g. between states, that can be estimated by the empirical transition matrix (ETM). Such multi-state models have had wide applications for modelling complex courses of a disease. In this chapter the ETM of multi-state and counting process (survival analytic) models which use the times for ICU patients to transition to varying states of violations (a violation being a carer's agitation rating outside so-called wavelet-probability bands (WPB)) confirm the utility of defining so-called trackers and non-trackers according to WPB-based control limits and rules. ETM and multi-state modelling demonstrate that these control-limit scoring approaches are suitable for developing more advanced optimal infusion controllers and coding of nurses A-S scores. These offer significant clinical potential of improved agitation management and reduced length of stay in critical care.

Keywords: agitation-sedation (A-S) control, nurses scores, empirical transition matrix (ETM), transition states, wavelet probability band (WPB)

1. Introduction

Pain management is increasingly recognised as a formal medical subspecialty worldwide [1]. Optimal sedation and analgesic strategies, combined with delirium management, are a challenge when caring for critically ill patients. Sedation in ICU aims to provide patient pain reflief, comfort and safety. For sedation monitoring, the most extensively used tools are RASS (Richmond Agitation and Sedation Scale) [2] and SAS (Sedation Agitation Scale) [3]. Despite extensive improvements in analgesia medication there are still barriers to nurses' assessment, management, documentation, and reassessment of pain [4–6].

Pain is the most common reason that patients come to the emergency department. Emergency nurses have an indispensable role in the management of this pain [7, 8]. Sedation in the intensive care unit (ICU) is challenging, as both over- and under-sedation are detrimental. Current methods of assessment, such as the Richmond Agitation Sedation Scale (RASS), are measured intermittently and invariable depend on patients' behavioural response to stimulation, as such may interrupt sleep and rest. A non-stimulating method for continuous sedation monitoring may be beneficial and allow more frequent assessment., noting that appropriate sedation cycling has to accommodate patients' oscillations between states of agitation and over-sedation, which are detrimental to patient health and increases hospital length of stay [9–14].

As such there also have been recent studies exploring the impact of augmenting sedation assessment with physiologic monitors [15] and studying the correlation between observational scales of sedation and bispectral index scores [16]. Recently the feasibility of continuous sedation monitoring of ICU patients using the NeuroSENSE was studied and suggested that such a non-stimulating method for continuous sedation monitoring may benefit patient care and allow increased A-S assessment [17]. The authors advocated use of incorporating some degree of automation into sedative drug administration, e.g. closed-loop control based on feedback from a processed EEG monitor, and various studies have suggested the limitations of RASS as a stand-alone measure of sedation levels, and pointed to benefit of adjunct continuous e.g., brain monitoring [17].

Earlier, Rudge, Chase, Shaw, Lee [12] discussed target controlled infusion (TCI) systems to deliver drugs to maintain target plasma concentrations, using a pharmacokinetic model, shown to be feasible when anaesthesia is given over short periods of reduced consciousness and well-known pharmacology is invoked. Infusion systems that regulate the infusion rate to maintain target agitation levels, to regulate the primary metric for longterm sedation, are one approach to improving care in the ICU. The data analysed in this chapter pertains to the scenario and data type studied earlier by [9–14].

Assessing the severity of agitation is a challenging clinical problem as variability related to drug metabolism for each individual is often subjective. A multitude of previous studies suggest that the assessment accuracy of the sedation quality conducted by nurses tend to suffer from subjectivity and lead to sub-optimal sedation [14, 15, 18]. For example, [19] strongly recommend lighter than deeper levels of sedations. Moreover, [20, 21] argue that sedation should be reviewed and adjusted regularly. Whilst agitation management methods frequently rely on subjective agitation assessment [2, 3] the carers then select an appropriate infusion rate based upon their evaluation of these scales, experience, and intuition [21]. This approach usually leads to largely continuous infusions which lack a bolus-focused approach, commonly resulting in over or under-sedation. The work of [11–13] aimed to enhance feedback protocols for medical decision support systems and eventually automated sedation administration. A minimal differential equation model to predict or simulate each patient's agitation-sedation status over time was presented in [12] for 37 ICU patients

	V1	V2	V3	Total V's	Time in ICU	WPB%
P18/Good	2	24	26	20	64	93.8%
P28/Poor	1	5	12	114	203	50.8%

Table 1.
Time to the patient-specific 1st violation V1, second violation V2 and third violation V3, total number of violations, total ICU time and WPB% values.

and was shown to capture patient A-S dynamics. The use of quantitative modelling to enhance understanding of the agitation-sedation (A-S) system and provision of an A-S simulation platform are one of the key tools in this area of patient critical care. A more refined A-S model, which utilised regression with an Epanechnikov kernel was formulated by [12]. A Bayesian approach using densities and wavelet shrinkage methods was later suggested by [9] to assess a previously derived deterministic, parametric A-S model [10–14], thus successfully challenging the practice of sedating ICU patients using continuous infusions. Wavelets approaches [9, 10] were shown to provide reliable diagnostics and visualisation tools to assess A-S models, giving alternative metrics of A-S control to assess validity of the earlier A-S deterministic models (**Table 1** in [10]).

This suite of wavelet metrics based on the discrete wavelet transform (DWT) were able to establish the value of earlier deterministic agitation-sedation (A-S) models against empirical (recorded) dynamic A-S infusion profiles, providing robust performance metrics of A-S control and excellent tools, as based on the classification of patients into poor and good trackers based on Wavelet Probability Bands (WPBs). Importantly, the WPBs were shown as a useful patient-specific method by which to identify and detect regions in the patient's A-S profile i.e., times whilst in ICU, where the simulated infusion rate performs poorly, thus providing visual and quantified ways to help improve and distil the deterministic A-S model and in practice be a guage to alert carers.

In this chapter Empirical Transition Matrix (ETM) approach of multi-state counting process (survival analytic) models of Allignol and coauthors [22, 23], aligned with the counting process/event history work in [24–26], which use the times patients transition to varying states of violations (a violation being an A-S measure outside the 90% WPB bands), confirm the utility of defining trackers and non-trackers according to these control limits and wavelet diagnostic rules of Kang et al., [9, 10]. In this chapter ETM and multi-state modelling are found to be valuable for developing advanced optimal infusion controllers and also to assist coding of nurses A-S scores, which potentially offer significant clinical potential of improved agitation management and reduced length of stay, as an augmented approach to also using RASS and SAS. Establishing patient-specific thresholds of poor A-S management and control has significant implications for the effective administration of sedatives, as improved management of A-S states will allow clinicians to improve the efficacy of care and reduce healthcare costs [27–29].

2. Data and methods

This chapter models the agitation-sedation profiles of Agitation and Sedation (A-S) profiles of 37 patients were collected at the Christchurch Hospital, Christchurch

School of Medicine and Health Sciences, NZ. Two measures were recorded for each patient: (1) the nurses' ratings of a patient's agitation level and (2) an automated sedation dose (see **Figure 1**). Infusion data were recorded using an electronic drug infusion device for all admitted ICU patients during a nine-month observation period and required more than 24 hours of sedation. Infusion data containing less than 48 hours of continuous data, or data from patients whose sedation requirements were extreme, such as those with severe head injuries, were excluded [9, 10]. A total of 37 ICU patients met these requirements and were enrolled in the study. Classification of patients into poor and good trackers, as based on the Wavelet Probability Bands (WPB) are given in **Table 2**. The so-called good tracker delineates the scenario where the nurse's rating scores remains within the (time based) 90% coverage of wavelet probability band (WPB) based on the simulated dose profiles [9, 10]. Poor tracking delineates the scenario where the nurses rating scores remain outside the (time based) 90% coverage of wavelet probability band (WPB) for a significant portion of time based on the simulated dose profiles [13, 14].

By way of illustration we consider four patients from the pool of 37 patients. **Tables 1** and **3** summarise each of these four patients' WPB tracker status, time to first, second and third violation outside the WPB bands [9], their total number of violations over ICU stay and patient's time in ICU, along with their specific WPB% value. Display of their line profiles of *nurses' rating* of A-S in relation to drug infusion *dose* over time, for each of the 4 patients (P8, P27, P18, P28) are given in **Figures 2–4**.

The first patient (patient 8) in **Table 3** is a good WPB tracker and the second a poor WPB tracker (patient 27), studied in depth in [28], for which upper tail thresholds of the nurses' scores using copulas were established. We also refer the reader also to Hudson & Tursunalieva's chapter in this book entitled "Copula thresholds and modelling Agitation-Sedation (A-S) in ICU: analysis of nurses scores of A-S and automated drug infusions by protocol" [27]. The corresponding WPB% values for patient 8 and patient 27 are 87.5% and 43.7%, respectively (**Table 3**). Overall, the minimum, median and maximum WPB% values for the 24 good trackers is (58.8%, 87.5%, 96.9%) and (47.3%, 64.8%, 77.3%) for the 13 poor trackers (**Table 2**). Noteworthy also is that the A-S time series of these two patients examined (P8 and P27) were of disparate lengths - patient eight had 10,561 time points and patient 27, 13,441 time points. The full 37 patients studied had a range of [3001–25,261] time points.

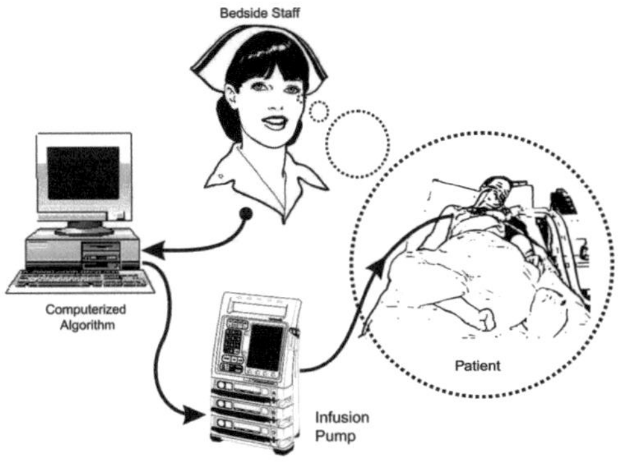

Figure 1.
Diagram of the feedback loop employing nursing staff's feedback of subjectively assessed patient agitation through the infusion controller (diagram is sourced from Chase et al. [14]).

WPB [9]	WCORR [10]	Chase et al. [14]	Rudge et al. [11]
2	2	—	—
4	4	—	—
—	—	6	—
7	7	7	7
9	9	9	
10	10	—	10
11	11	—	11
—	—	12	—
—	—	—	13
—	—	17	—
21	21	21	—
22	22	—	22
27	27	27	27
28	28	—	28
—	29	—	29
32	32	—	—
33	33	—	33
34	34	34	—
—	35	—	35
Total: N_1 = 13	Total: N_2 = 15	Total: N_3 = 8	Total: N_4 = 10

Table 2.
Patient numbers of the ***poor*** *trackers according to the criteria of 4 studies. Developed earlier in [11–14]. Low WPB 90% indicates a poor tracker by Kang's WPB diagnostics [9, 10].*

	V1	V2	V3	Total V's	Time in ICU	WPB%
P8/Good	1	2	3	46	128	87.5%
P27/Poor	1	4	5	89	225	43.7%

Table 3.
Time to the patient-specific 1st violation V1, second violation V2 and third violation V3, total number of violations, total ICU time and WPB% values.

Patient 18 (good tracker) with a WPB% of 93.8% and patient 28 (poor tracker) with WPB% of 50.8% (**Table 1**) were studied in detail in [28], for which both upper and lower tails/thresholds of over or under-estimation of agitation levels by the nurses rating were established using copula dependence analytics [29], refer also to [27].

Patients vary according to their length of stay in ICU and consequently differ in their opportunity for violations to occur. The good trackers generally have shorter ICU time and thus less chance to exibit an increased total number of violations. An indication of how the strata (good versus poor tracker), the patient's total number of violations and a patient's time in ICU interact, can be visualied in **Figure 5**. The total number of WPB based violations is clearly greater for the poor trackers than for the

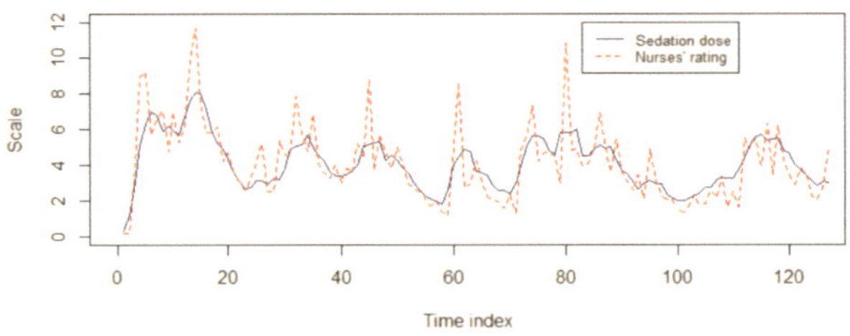

Figure 2.
Line plot of nurses' rating of patient agitation and the automated sedation dose for patient 8 (good tracker).

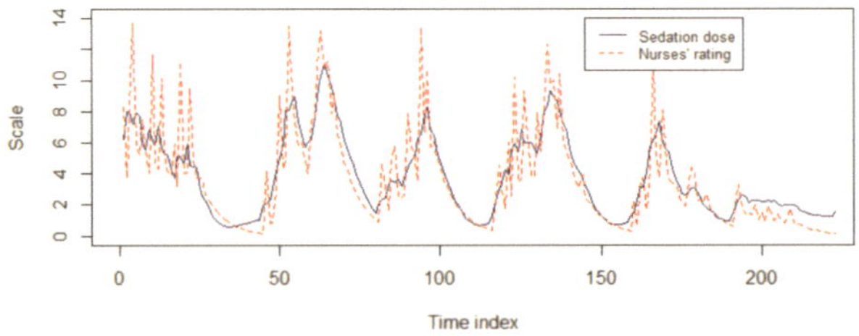

Figure 3.
Line plot of nurses' rating of patient agitation and the automated sedation dose for patient 27 (good tracker).

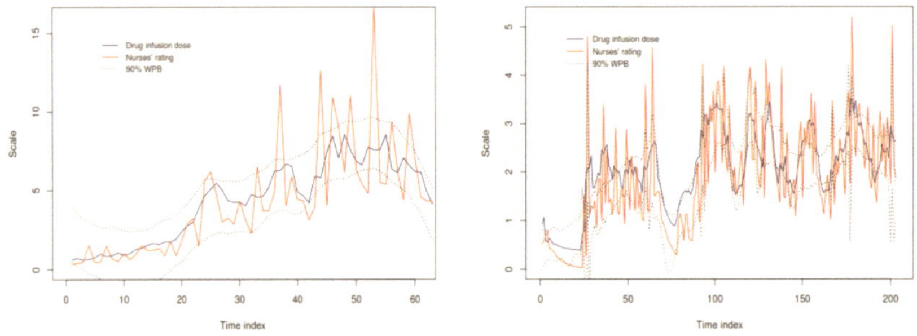

Figure 4.
Line plot and WPB% band for patient 18 (LHS) and 28 (RHS, poor tracker).

good trackers, and it is the poor trackers that tend to have longer ICU times. Also from the scatterplot in **Figure 5** there seems to be three approximate categories of patient ICU time: 50–64, 113–128 and 205–256. The majority of patients (28 (76%)) have ≤40 violations (RHS of **Figure 5**), 19 (51%) patients have an ICU time of ≤64 (**Table 4**).

Accordingly, for ICU time categorised and coded as: 0 = [50,64], 1 = [113,128], and 2 = [205,256], the total violations profile according to tracking status, displayed in **Figure 6**, shows that the total number of violations is significantly higher for the poor trackers, particularly when ICU time > 205. Noteworthy, is that the majority of patients 28 (76%) have ≤40 violations (RHS of **Figure 6**), whereas 19 (51%) patients have an ICU time ≤ 64 (**Table 4**). **Figure** 7 displays the histogram of the number of violations where a violation is defined as a nurse's A-S rating outside the patient's WPB control band. We note that the majority of the time, in excess of >75% of the 370 violation counts are below a count of five violations (**Figure** 7).

DOI: http://dx.doi.org/10.5772/intechopen.105480

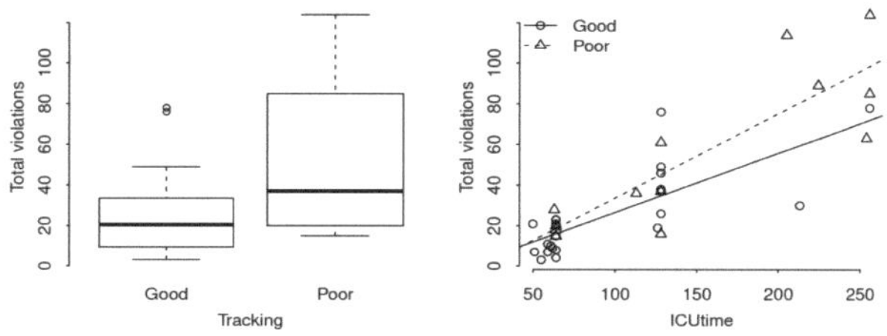

Figure 5.
Total number of violations by WPB tracking status [9] and ICU time.

	ICU category		
WPB tracker	**0**	**1**	**2**
Good	15	7	2
Poor	4	4	5

Table 4.
Patient tracker status by ICU time: 0 = 50–64, 1 = 113–128, 2 = 205–256.

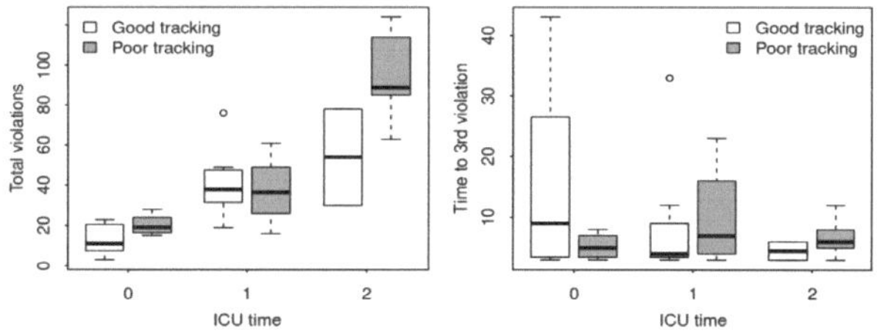

Figure 6.
Total number of violations by 3 levels of ICU time (LHS) and boxplot of poor good tracker time to 3rd violation by ICU time: 0 = [50,64], 1 = [113,128], 2 = [205,256].

For the state-space analysis described in Section 3 each patient's total ICU time is broken into 10 bins, where each bin represents 10% of the patients' total time in ICU; i.e., Bin 1: 0–10%, Bin 2: 11–20% etc. For the 37 patients, we thus have 370 bins, i.e. 370 counts of violations. The 10% interval approach is used due to the large variation in time in ICU between the WPB-based good versus poor strata [9] - noting that some poor trackers have times up to 256, whereas good trackers are mostly limited to 64–128. Given these bins, patients' A-S states can then be defined in terms of the total number of violations or jumps outside the WPB bands that occur during each 10% interval of a patient's total ICU time. The randon, outcome event of A-S status is then the number of violations that over time.

3. Empirical transition matrix state-space & commenges' test approach

3.1 Mathematical formulation

Multi-state models are known to provide a relevant framework for modelling complex event histories. Quantities of interest are mainly the transition probabilities

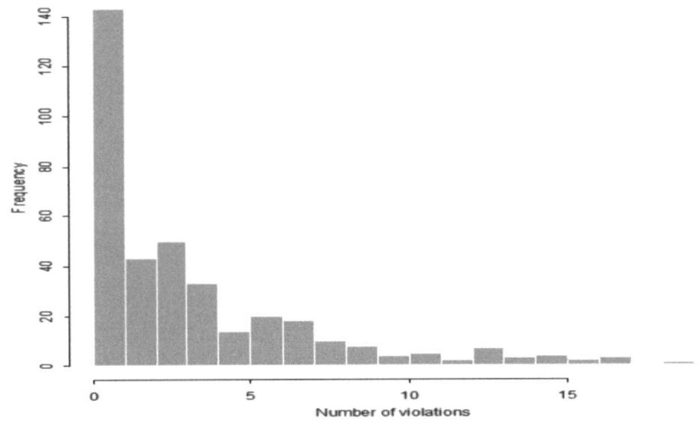

Figure 7.
Violation counts in bins across all patients.

that can be estimated by the empirical transition matrix, that is also referred to as the Aalen-Johansen estimator [30, 31]. Such multi-state models have had a wide range of applications for modelling complex courses of a disease over the course of time and across applications in medical research (Beyersmann et al. [32], Munoz-Price et al. [33], Andersen & Keiding [34]). We now utilise the Empirical Transition Matrix (etm) approach to model multi-state models of [22] and derive inference tests for such models using the approach of Commenges [25, 35, 36] with a particular focus on Commenges' test derived in earlier work [25].

Define patient states as follows, any state can transition into any other state (**Figure 8**).

- State 1: 0 or 1 violations
- State 2: 2 or 3 violations
- State 3: > 3 violations

A number of different approaches (etm on ICU time, etm on bin time, and log-rank type tests as in Commenges [25], will be used to investigate the difference between good and poor trackers in terms of a devised a 3 state transition formulation as defined below. Differences between transition probabilities between states for the good and poor trackers will be evaluated using Commenges' [25] chi square test.

The mathematics is well described in the work of Allignol [22], adapted to more complex scenarios in [23]; and in Commenges' approach [25, 35, 36]. The mathematical formulation of the ETM state-space approach and Commenges' test are given for general frameworks as follows.

Consider a stochastic process (X_t) with finite state space $S = \{1, \ldots, K\}$ where sample paths are right-continuous, and the stochastic process is assumed to be

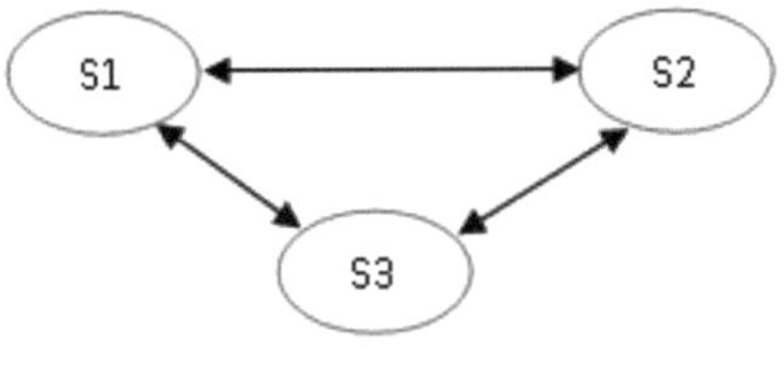

Figure 8.
State-space system.

time-inhomogeneous Markov. The transition hazard from state i to state j, $i \neq j$ is defined as

$$\alpha_{ij}(t)dt = P(X_{t+dt} = j \mid X_t = i).$$

The cumulative hazard transitions are defined as,

$$A_{ij}(t) = \int_0^t \alpha_{ij}(t)dt$$
$$A_{ii}(t) = -\sum_{j \neq i} A_{ij}(t).$$

Define

$$P_{ij}(s,t) = P(X_t = j \mid X_s = i), \text{for } i,j \in S, s \leq t$$

as the probability that an individual who is in state i at time s is in state j at time t.

The (K + 1)x(K + 1) probability transition matrix with elements $P_{ij}(s,t)$ can then be obtained from the transition hazards through product integration. Let $N_{ij}(t)$ be the number of observed direct transitions from state I to state j up to time t and let $Y_i(t)$ be the number of individuals under observation in state I just before time t. The Nelson-Aalen estimator is used to estimate the non-diagonal elements of the matrix of cumulative hazards as follows,

$$\hat{A}_{ij}(t) = \int_0^t \frac{dN_{ij}(u)}{Y_i(u)}, i \neq j$$

and the diagonal elements $\hat{A}_{ii}(t)$ are obtained as above. The product integration relationship below leads to an estimate of the probability transition matrix as follows,

$$\hat{\boldsymbol{P}}(s,t) = \prod_{s < t_k \leq t} \left(\boldsymbol{I} + \Delta \hat{\boldsymbol{A}}(t_k) \right),$$

where the product is taken over all possible transition times in time interval (s,t].

An estimator for the covariance of the empirical transition matrix is given by,

$$\widehat{\text{cov}}\left(\hat{\boldsymbol{P}}(s,t)\right) = \int_s^t \hat{\boldsymbol{P}}(u,t)^T \otimes \hat{\boldsymbol{P}}(s,u-) \widehat{\text{cov}}\left(d\hat{\boldsymbol{A}}(u)\right) \hat{\boldsymbol{P}}(u,t) \otimes \hat{\boldsymbol{P}}(s,u-),^T$$

which is a $(K + 1)^2$ x $(K + 1)^2$ matrix, with number or rows and columns equal $(K + 1)^2$.

3.2 Commenges' test formulation

We now utilise the framework of the generalised Cochran–Mantel–Haenszel (CMH) test for (I x J x K) tables. The CMH test is based on the hypergeometric distribution. The CMH and the test of Commenges' for the specific case here, where we have three states (of violations) and two strata (good versus poor trackers) is now described.

In our application then we have $2 \times 3 \times 3$ tables. For each k = 1, 2, 3 we have a 2×3 table, where the elements are counts n_{ijk} (k denotes the departure state j, so the rows, I, are the WPB strata, the columns, J, are the entry states I and the slices, K, are the departure states j), as tabulated below.

	I = 0	I = 1	I = 2	Row total
Good	n_{11k}	n_{12k}	n_{13k}	n_{1+k}
Poor	n_{21k}	n_{22k}	n_{23k}	n_{2+k}
Total	n_{+1k}	n_{+2k}	n_{+3k}	n_{++k}

Assume that the row and column marginals are fixed. This implies that there are (I-1) by (J-1) values that are free to vary. For the cell n_{ijk} the expected value is then given by n_{i+k} x n_{+jk}. We are able to express all cell counts by the vector $\mathbf{n_k}$ and express all expected cell counts by $\mathbf{u_k}$. The covariance matrix, denoted by $\mathbf{V_k}$ then has elements,

$$cov\left(n_{ijk}, n_{i'j'k}\right) = \frac{n_{i+k}(\delta_{ii'}n_{++k} - n_{i'+k})n_{+jk}\left(\delta_{jj'}n_{++k} - n_{+j'k}\right)}{n^2_{++k}(n_{++k} - 1)},$$

where $\delta_{ab} = 1$ when a = b, and 0 otherwise. Assuming rows and columns are unordered we sum over the K strata to obtain,

$$n = \sum n_k, \quad u = \sum u_k, \quad V = \sum V_k.$$

The generalised CMH statistic is then given by,

$$X^2 = (\boldsymbol{n} - \boldsymbol{u})'^{V^{-1}}(\boldsymbol{n} - \boldsymbol{u}),$$

which follows a chi square distribution with (I-1) by (J-1) degrees of freedom. This test is implemented in R via the mantelhaen.test function. Commenges [25] adapts this concept, with a test which differs to the generalised CMH test in that it does not sum over the K strata, before calculating the relevant chi squared test statistic.

Commenges' test [25] is as follows,

$$X_k^2 = (\boldsymbol{n_k} - \boldsymbol{u_k})'^{V^{-1}}(\boldsymbol{n_k} - \boldsymbol{u_k}),$$

where X_k^2 is chi-square with (I-1) by (J-1) degrees of freedom.

The required total chi squared statistic is then simply obtained by taking $X^2 = \sum X_k^2$ which is itself disctributed as a chi square distribution with K(I-1) by (J-1) degrees of freedom.

3.3 Results of the ETM analysis and Commenges' test on transition states

Conditionally on the number of patients in each state at each step we have 3 x 9 = 27 independent contingency tables (i.e., number of departure states j by the number of time points k–1, recall we have 10, 10% bins for a patient's time in ICU) and each of these tables has dimension 2 × 3 (good/poor tracker by the number of states i).

The corresponding three specific strata tables are given in **Tables 5–7**. For example, for departure state j = 0 and time point k = 2 we have a two by three contingency table with an overall total of 7^{Φ} violations (labelled $^{\Phi}$ in **Table 5**); the latter informs that, at time k = 2 there are 5^{Φ} good WPB based trackers that depart from state j = 0

	Strata	I = 0	I = 1	I = 2	Total
k = 2	Good	5^{Φ}	0	0	5
	Poor	0	2^{Φ}	0	2
	Total	5	2	0	7^{Φ}
k = 3	Good	10	5	1	16
	Poor	0	1	0	1
	Total	10	6	1	17
k = 4	Good	10	1	0	11
	Poor	2	0	0	2
	Total	12	1	0	13
k = 5	Good	9	2	2	13
	Poor	0	3	1	4
	Total	9	5	3	17
k = 6	Good	9	3	2	14
	Poor	0	0	0	0
	Total	9	3	2	14
k = 7	Good	9	2	2	13
	Poor	1	1	0	2
	Total	10	3	2	15
k = 8	Good	5	4	2	11
	Poor	2	0	2	4
	Total	7	4	4	15
k = 9	Good	5	2	0	7
	Poor	3	0	0	3
	Total	8	2	0	10
k = 10	Good	9	1	1	11
	Poor	2	1	2	5
	Total	11	2	3	16

Table 5.
Departure state j = 0: WPB strata [9].

and enter state 0. Similarly there are two (2^{Φ}) WPB based poor trackers that depart state j = 0 and enter state 1 (**Table 5**).

Three 2 x 3 contingency tables (one for each departure state j) are thus created.

Estimated transition probabilities for the 3 state process are then plotted using the 'xyplot' function from the lattice package in R. In the resultant plots (**Figures 9–11**), the vertical y-axis represents the transition probability value, which is represented by the solid line in each plot region. The numbers in the coloured bar above each plot defines the transition (e.g., 1 2 means transition probability from state 1 to state 2). The dotted lines around the solid line represent the confidence bands based on the covariance as calculated by the etm function. The horizontal x-axis shows the the

	Strata	I = 0	I = 1	I = 2	Total
k = 2	Good	6	1	1	8
	Poor	1	1	0	2
	Total	7	2	1	10
k = 3	Good	1	2	0	3
	Poor	2	2	2	6
	Total	3	4	2	9
k = 4	Good	2	2	3	7
	Poor	2	2	0	4
	Total	4	4	3	11
k = 5	Good	3	1	1	5
	Poor	0	1	2	3
	Total	3	2	3	8
k = 6	Good	3	1	0	4
	Poor	1	3	1	5
	Total	4	4	1	9
k = 7	Good	2	3	1	6
	Poor	3	2	0	5
	Total	5	5	1	11
k = 8	Good	2	2	3	7
	Poor	1	1	2	4
	Total	3	3	5	11
k = 9	Good	4	3	2	9
	Poor	0	1	0	1
	Total	4	4	2	10
k = 10	Good	4	1	2	7
	Poor	1	1	0	2
	Total	5	2	2	9

Table 6.
Departure state j = 1: WPB strata [9].

time i.e., 10% bins (i.e. 2–10, because no transitions occur at time one being the initial state). For each tracker status and possible piairs of state transitions there are three plots, given in the following order, good trackers, poor trackers. **Figure 11** displays the probability of being in each of the 3 states (0, 1, 2) given the initial state is state 0.

Our procedure results in three 2 x 3 contingency tables (one for each departure state j), see **Tables 8–10**. The chi squared statistic as derived in [25] can now be calculated in that for the Commenges test the same chi squared calculation is made for each state specific table separately (i.e., without summing over k). The results in this case are $\chi^2(1) = 6.046$, $\chi^2\ (2) = 2.269$ and $\chi^2(3) = 9.280$. Each of these follows a chi

	Strata	I = 0	I = 1	I = 2	Total
k = 2	Good	5	2	4	11
	Poor	0	3	6	9
	Total	5	5	10	20
k = 3	Good	0	0	5	5
	Poor	0	1	5	6
	Total	0	1	10	11
k = 4	Good	1	2	3	6
	Poor	0	1	6	7
	Total	1	3	9	13
k = 5	Good	2	1	3	6
	Poor	0	1	5	6
	Total	2	2	8	12
k = 6	Good	1	2	3	6
	Poor	1	2	5	8
	Total	2	4	8	14
k = 7	Good	0	2	3	5
	Poor	0	1	5	6
	Total	0	3	8	11
k = 8	Good	0	3	3	6
	Poor	0	0	5	5
	Total	0	3	8	11
k = 9	Good	2	2	4	8
	Poor	2	1	6	9
	Total	4	3	10	17
k = 10	Good	2	1	3	6
	Poor	1	0	5	6
	Total	3	1	8	12

Table 7.
Departure state $j = 2$: WPB strata [9].

square distribution with 2 degrees of freedom with associated p-values of 0.049, 0.322 and 0.010 (**Table 11**). Kang WPB (2013) [9].

Summing these three $\chi^2(j)$, j = 1,2,3 statistics gives a value of $\chi^2 = 17.59$ with 6 degrees of freedom and an associated p-value of 0.007 (**Table 11**). The underlying null hypothesis is that the two nominal variables (strata: good or poor tracker and entry state: 0, 1, or 2) are conditionally independent in each stratum (departure state j; 0, 1 or 2), assuming no three-way interaction. The low p-value of 0.007 suggests that this hypothesis be rejected, i.e., the two variables are not conditionally independent. Thus the Commenges test shows that there is a statistically significant difference between the good versus poor tracker WPB strata, and that this difference is mainly

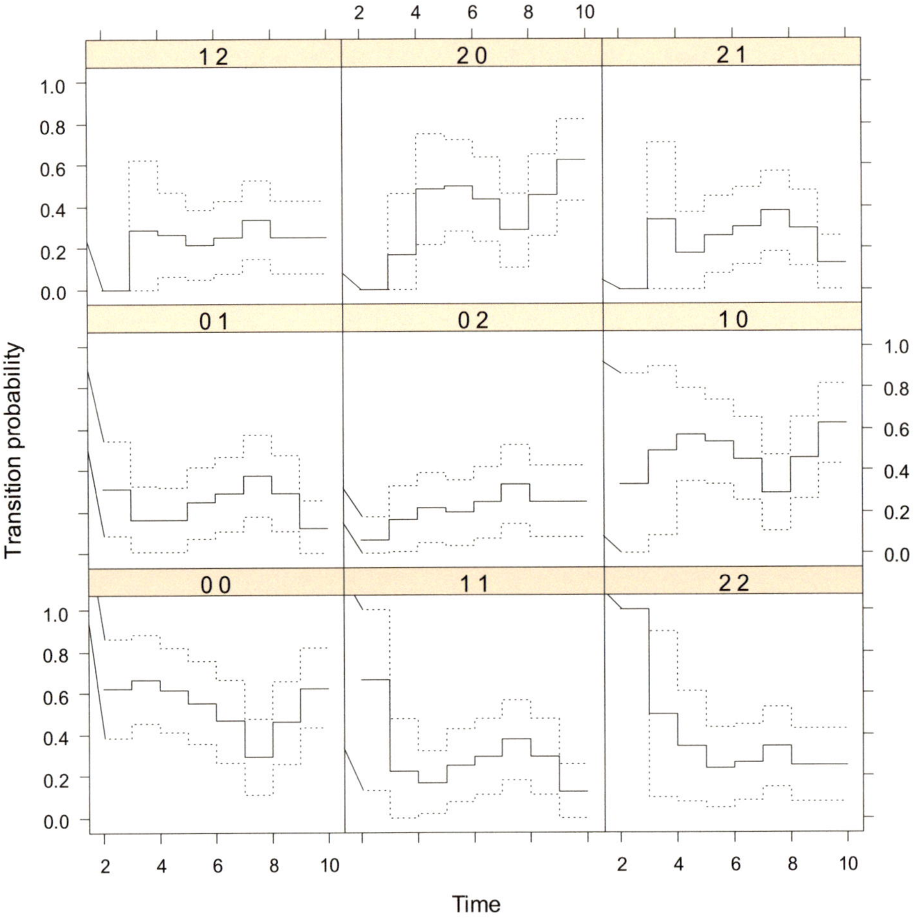

Figure 9.
Transition probability profiles for WPB good trackers.

due to transitions out of states 0 and 2, which agrees with the trends based on a graphical inspection of **Figures 9–11**.

The same procedure and related Commenges' test is then applied to each of the 3 remaining good/poor tracker definitions of Kang [10, 11, 14] for the three-state context studied in this chapter. These results are reported in **Table 12**.

Kang et al., WCORR [10].

Chase et al. [14].

State	χ^2	p-value
J = 0	5.669	0.059
J = 1	6.406	**0.041***
J = 2	3.097	0.213
Total	**15.172**	**0.019****

Rudge et al. [11].

State	χ^2	p-value
J = 0	0.367	0.832
J = 1	2.951	0.229
J = 2	5.466	0.065*
Total	**8.784**	0.186

Transition probability profiles of being in each state as time progresses, given start state 0, for the remaining 3 studies of [10, 14, 11] are given in **Figures 12–14**. In summary, **Figures 9–14** illustrate the trend that good trackers tend to have higher probability of transitioning into state 0 than poor trackers, and the good trackers tend to have lower probability of transitioning into state two than poor trackers, where state two indicates that more violations (>3 violations) are occurring, and state 0 indicates few violations are occurring.

Notably also, the probability of transitioning into state 2 overall appears to increase as ICU time increases. This is most likely because poor tracking patients tend to have longer ICU times, and so, as time goes on, it is only poor trackers transitions that are being estimated. By categorising patients according to total ICU time (≤64, >64) as discussed earlier (**Figures 5** and **6**, **Table 4**) some of this could be accounted for. The results obtained are still consistent, as shown in the etm profiles using ICU time (≤64, >64) in **Figures 15** and **16**, respectively. The corresponding ETM probabilities are determined according to etm in R [21] and associated state and strata specific plots given in **Figures 15** and **16**.

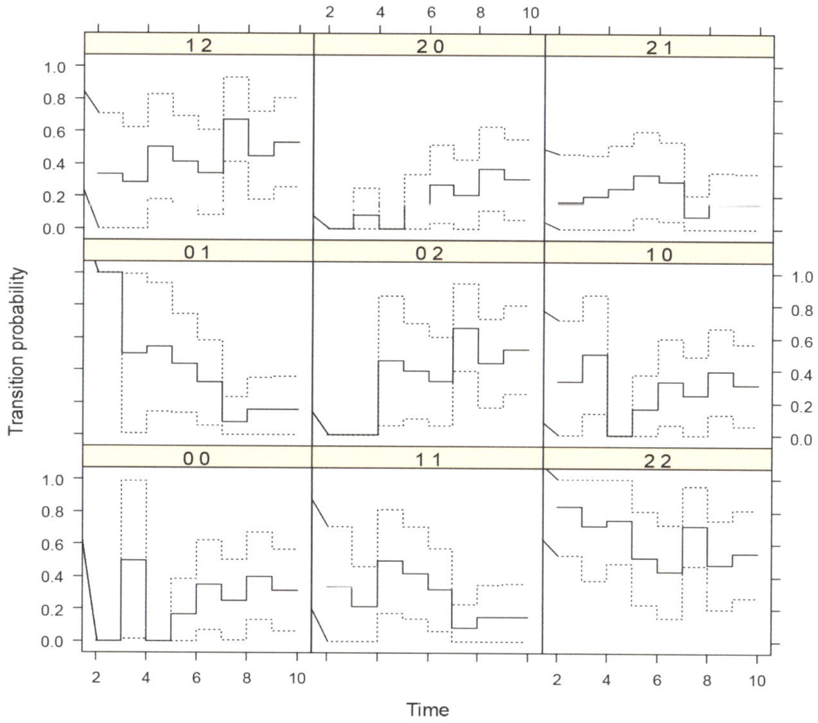

Figure 10.
Transition probability profiles for WPB poor trackers.

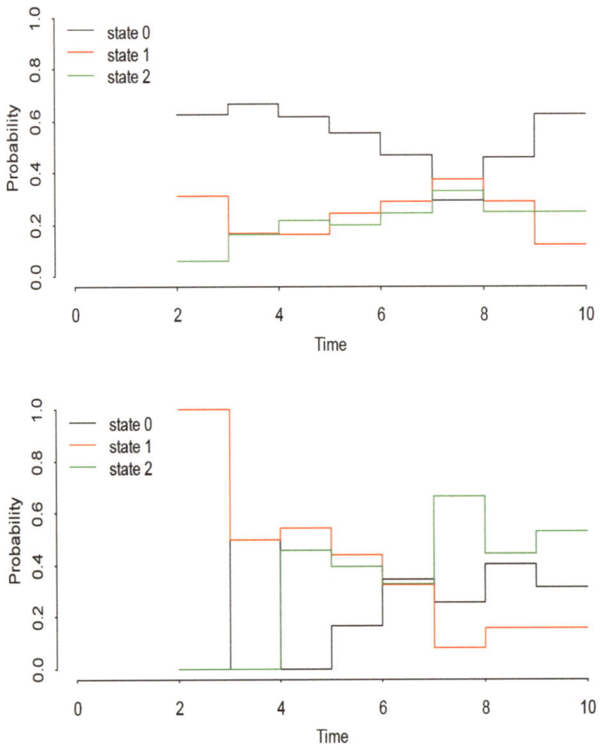

Figure 11.
Probability of being in each state as time progresses given start state 0. Top is good trackers, bottom is poor trackers: WPB based.

Tracker strata	I = 0	I = 1	I = 2	Total
Good	71	20	10	101
Poor	10	8	5	23
Total	81	28	15	124

Table 8.
Departure state $j = 0$ summed over all time points k, $k = 2, \ldots, 10$.

Tracker strata	I = 0	I = 1	I = 2	Total
Good	27	16	13	56
Poor	11	14	7	32
Total	38	30	20	88

Table 9.
Departure state $j = 1$ summed over all time points k, $k = 2, \ldots, 10$.

3.4 Conclusion regarding the ETM based analysis

The different approaches in Section 3 led to the sasimilar conclusions that there is a difference in the way good trackers and poor trackers transition between states. Most

Tracker strata	I = 0	I = 1	I = 2	Total
Good	13	15	31	59
Poor	4	10	48	62
Total	17	25	79	121

Table 10.
Departure state $j = 2$ summed over all time points k, $k = 2, \ldots, 10$.

State	χ^2	p-value
J = 0	6.046	**0.049***
J = 1	2.269	0.322
J = 2	9.280	**0.010****
Total	**17.59**	**0.007*****

Table 11.
Computation of Commenges' test for the WPB strata [9].

State	χ^2	p-value
J = 0	1.724	0.422
J = 1	0.911	0.634
J = 2	7.123	**0.028****
Total	**9.758**	0.135

Table 12.
Computation of Commenges' test for the remaining A-S studies.

of this difference occurs in states 0 and states 2, as defined. Good trackers tend to have higher probability of transitioning into state 0 than poor trackers, and good trackers tend to have lower probability of transitioning into state 2 than poor trackers, noting that state 2 indicates more violations are occurring, and state 0 indicates fewer violations. The probability of transitioning into state 2 overall appears to increase as ICU time increases. This is most likely due to the fact that poor tracking patients have longer ICU times, and so, as time goes on, it is only the poor trackers' transitions that are being estimated.

By categorising patients according to their total ICU time (≤ 64, >64) similar trends were found. The Commenges' test established a statistically significant difference between the two tracking strata ($p = 0.007$), and that this difference was mainly due to transitions out of states 0 and 2. For the tracking metric of Chase et al. [14], the Commenges test demonstrated a statistically significant difference between the two good versus poor strata ($p = 0.019$), with this difference mainly due to transitions out of states 0 and 1. Overall, the WCORR [10] and Rudge [11] classifications of tracking/strata, the transision probability profiles for the 3 state process, good and poor trackers are not significantly different, but exhibited some difference mainly due to transitions out of state 2.

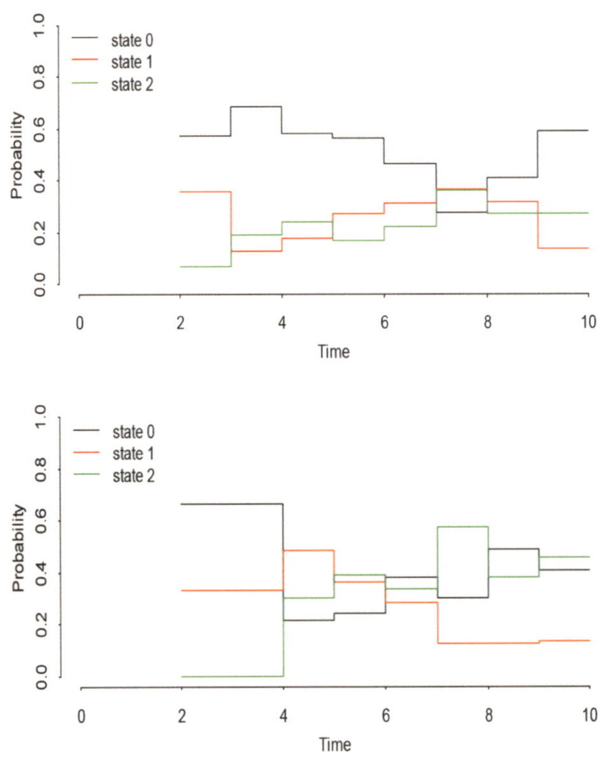

Figure 12.
Probability of being in each state as time progresses given start state 0. Top is good trackers; bottom is poor trackers: WCORR of [10].

4. Time-to-response bias as a counting process mult state model

4.1 Mathematical formulation

In this section we analyse the WPB violation data and investigate the times to the third violation given times to second violation for both poor trackers and good trackers where tracking status is defined by WPB diagnostics. The process can be thought to have three states. State 1 corresponds to less than two violations, state 2 means two violations and if a patient is in state 3 then three violations have occurred. This is a sequential three state process shown schematically in **Figure 17**. Events of interest are a transition from state 2 to state 3, i.e. the occurrence of a third violation.

Time one is the patient's entry time into state 2 and time two is the patients exit time from state 2 (i.e., entry time to state 3, so-called 'death' state). Time one is the patient's entry time into state 2 and time two is the patient's exit time from state 2 (i.e., entry time to state 3, so-called 'death' state).

In the case of multiple events of interest, the process can be treated as a Markov chain. Let N_{ij} (t) be the process counting the number of observed transitions from state i to state j in the interval [0, t]. The transition intensity from state i to state j at time t is then λ_{ij} (t) and gives the instantaneous risk of transition from state i to j.

N_{ij} (t) has intensity process of the form $\lambda_{ij}(t)N_i(t)$ where $Y_i(t)$ is the number of individuals in state i just before time t. This is the setup of Simon and Makuch [37] who considered 4 states and two transitions of interest.

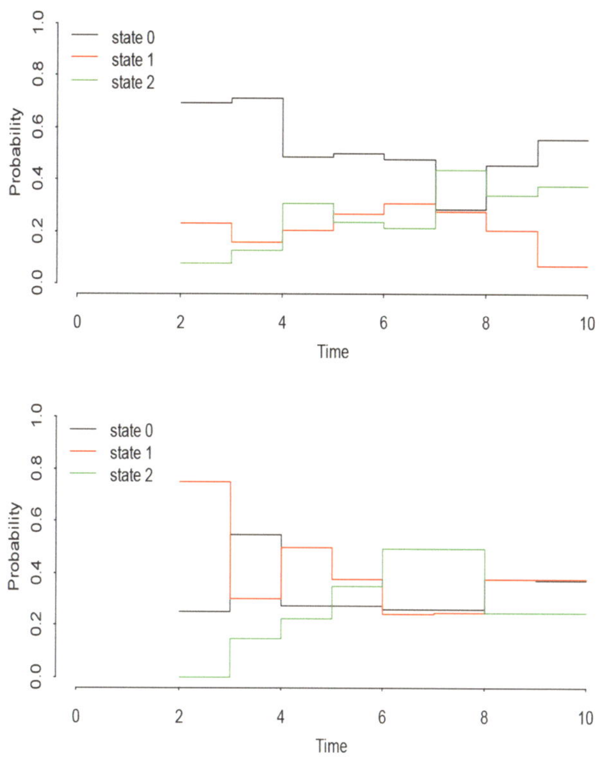

Figure 13.
Probability of being in each state as time progresses given start state 0. Top is good trackers; bottom is poor trackers according to Chase et al. [14].

The concept of time in our ICU application represents time on-study (i.e. time at ICU) rather than calendar time. In the case of our 3 state process (**Figure 8**) the hazard functions of the two transitions of interest are $\lambda_{13}(t)$ and $\lambda_{23}(t)$ and the number of individuals in the states just before t are $N_1(t)$ and N_2 (t), respectively. A chi squared test is conducted to test for independence between response and non-response as in the development formulated in [37].

This same test can be conducted to assess the association between strata and hazard rate. If $\lambda_{23}(0)(t)$ is the hazard rate (from state 2 to 3) for the good trackers and $\lambda_{23}(1)$ is the hazard rate (from state 2 to 3) for the poor tackers. Since the focus here is to test the effect of response (prior 2nd violation) on the hazard function, the null hypothesis of interest is H_0: $\lambda_{23}(0)$ (t) = $\lambda_{23}(1)$. The hypothesis is tested via a log-rank type test following [37] which tests for the time-to-response bias. Now the equivalent of **Table 2** in Simon and Makuch [37] can be constructed for both the good trackers and the poor trackers. Let $N_1(t)$ be the number of patients in state 1 at time t, and let N_2 (t) denote the number of patients in state 2 at time t in **Table 13**.

Table 13 presents the WPB data as state-specific patient counts for each event time t. *Events are a transition from state 2 to state 3,* i.e. the occurrence of the event of interest i.e. a third violation. Time represents time to third violation (so-called end-state/death in terms of a counting process). Note that d_{ij} (t) are the so-called end-state "deaths" i.e., third violations. The hazard function for transfers between states i and j at time t is denoted by $\lambda_{i\,j}$ (t) and here time represents time on study at ICU. Also T_{ij} denotes

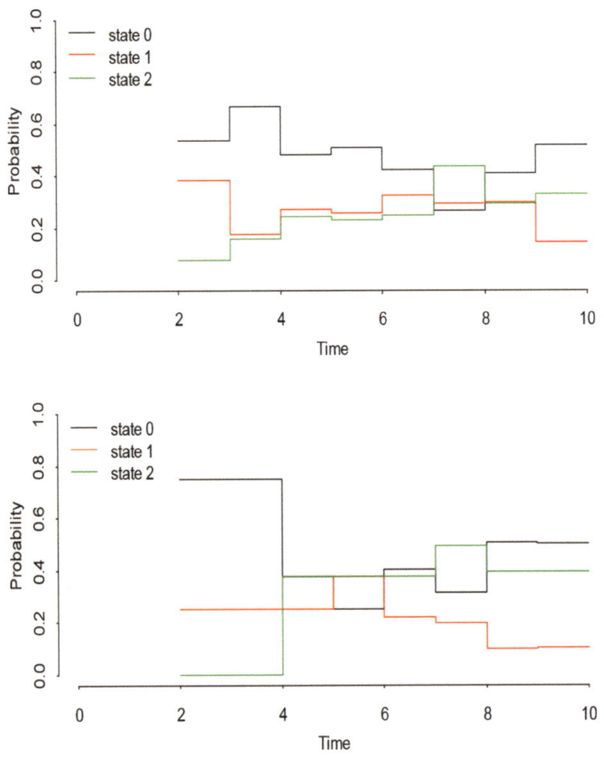

Figure 14.
Probability of being in each state as time progresses given start state 0. Top is good trackers; bottom is poor trackers according to Rudge et al. [11].

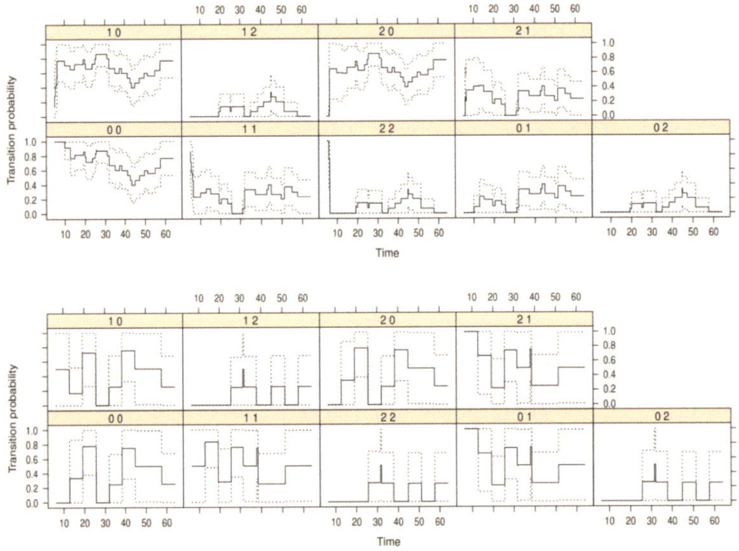

Figure 15.
Transition probability profiles for patients with ICU time ≤ 64. Top panel are the WPB good trackers, and bottom panel the poor trackers.

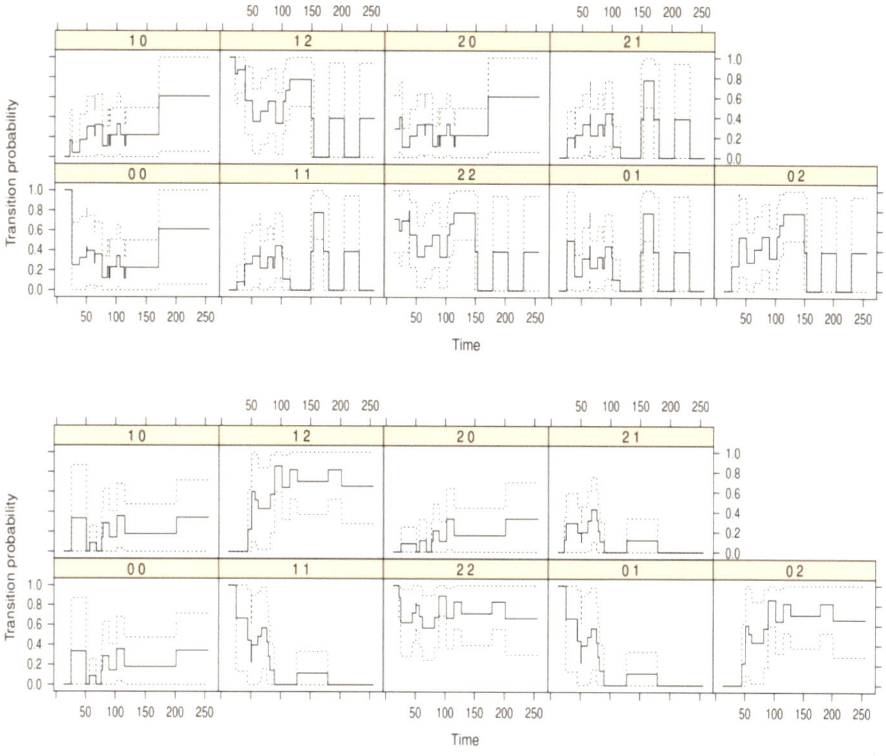

Figure 16.
Transition probability profiles for patients with ICU time > 64. Top panel are the WPB good trackers, and bottom panel the poor trackers.

the set of times at which a transition from state i to state j occurs and $N_i(t)$ is the number of patients in state i just before time t, or in other words, $N_i(t)$ is the number of patients at risk of a transfer out of state i at time t. (Note our Ni (t) is equivalent to $Y_i(t)$ in the Aalen's notation). The symbol λ_{ij} (t) denotes the intensity, or hazard function, for a transfer from state i to state j at time t.

Mathematically the cumulative hazard function is conventionally estimated instead of the hazard function $\lambda(t)$, as the latter is difficult to estimate. The cumulative hazard function and survival function is then given as,

$$\hat{A}_{ij}(x,t) = \sum -\log\left(1 - d_{ij}(u)/N_i(u)\right)$$
$$\hat{S}_{ij}(x,t) = \prod\left(1 - d_{ij}(u)/N_i(u)\right)$$
$$= \exp\left(-\hat{A}_{ij}(x,t)\right)$$

Note that $d_{ij}(u)$ above are the so-called end-state "deaths" i.e., third violations, the number of transitions from state i to state j in time interval [x, t]. The estimated survival and cumulative hazard curves are shown as in **Figure 18.**

Survival curves and cumulative hazard functions were calculated according to Simon and Makuch's method [37]. In essence, this counting process formulation keeps track of the number of patients in state 1 and 2 and event times (i.e., transitions into state 3). The survival package is used for estimation, where two times are used. Time

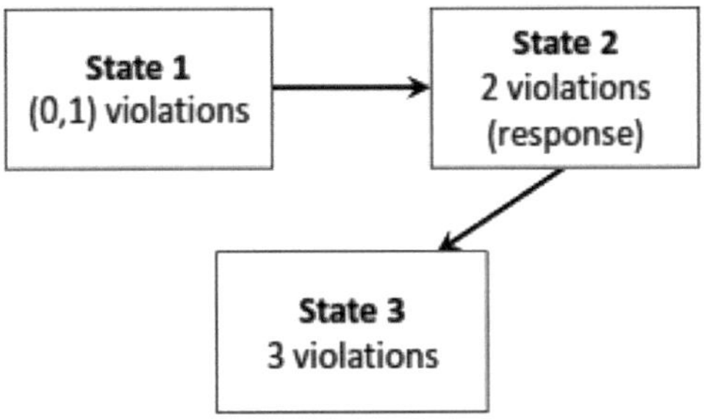

Figure 17.
States of a patient's agitation (violations) defined by certain levels of violations or jumps outside of the patient's WPB bands - a 3 state process.

Time	N_1	N_2	Events
3	12	12	7
4	7	10	5
6	6	6	2
9	5	5	1
12	4	5	1
18	2	6	1
19	2	5	1
26	0	6	1
27	0	5	1
28	0	4	1
33	0	3	1
36	0	2	1
43	0	1	1

(a) Good trackers.

Time	N_1	N_2	Events
3	9	4	3
4	8	2	1
5	5	4	2
6	3	4	2
8	1	4	2
9	1	2	1
12	1	1	1
23	0	1	1

(b) Poor trackers

Table 13.
Simon and Makuch's [37] represeantation and formulation of the WPB data.

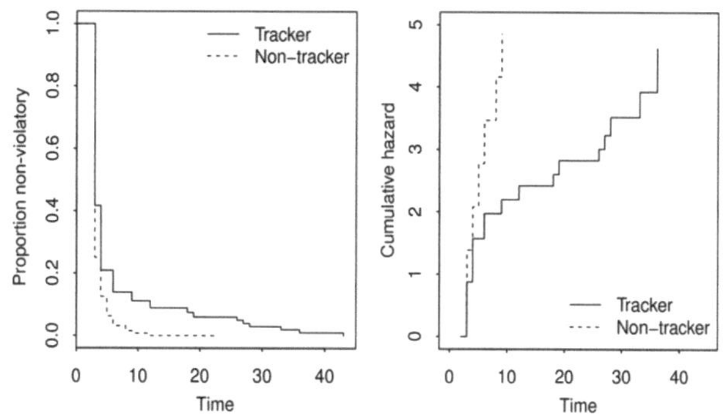

Figure 18.
Survival function of time to 3rd violation given the 2nd violation for good tracker and poor (non-)trackers (LHS) and cumulative hazard functions (RHS).

one is the patients entry time into state 2 and time two is the patients exit time from state 2 (i.e. entry time to state 3, 'death').

The log rank test for H_0: $\lambda_{23}(0)$ (t) = $\lambda_{23}(1)$, based on the counting process which utilises the number of individuals in the states just before t, these are, $N_1(t)$ and N_2 (t), was performed. Accordingly, it is shown that the good tracker and poor tracker hazard rates/ (survival curves) time to the 3rd violation, given a 2nd violation has occurred, are statistically significantly different (p-value = 0.044), see left hand side of **Figure 18**. Notably, the hazard rate for the poor trackers is 2.1 times that of good trackers, 95% confidence interval (CI) [1.01, 4.38].

Further interpretation of the hazard function can be made by assessing the slope of the cumulative hazard function. **Figure 18** (RHS), shows that the cumulative hazard increases faster for the poor trackers than the good trackers indicated by a much steeper slope. This suggests it takes less time for the poor trackers to reach their third violation than for the good trackers, this is also confirmed by the 95% confidence bands for the survival curves shown in **Figure 19** for the good tracker and poor trackers. Note that the interpretation of Kaplan–Meier curves here is not as straight-forward as for conventional survival analysis. In our ICU A-S process formulation the curves do not correspond to fixed cohorts, as patients can contribute to different states/curves at different times (**Table 13**). Thereby the curves may be

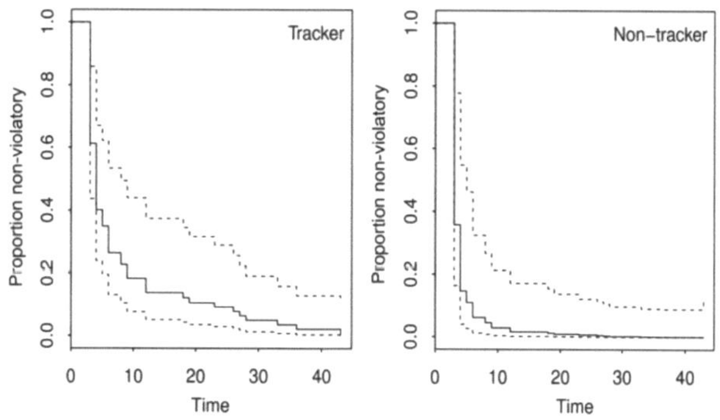

Figure 19.
Survival curves (95% CIs) for good (left) and poor (right) (non-)trackers.

considered to represent hypothetical cohorts whose values remain constant after follow-up [38, 39].

A Cox proportional hazards model (CPHM) was then fitted with tracking status and a patient's number of violations as covariates. The general CPHM hazard function is,

$$\lambda(\mathrm{t}|X) = \lambda_0 \exp\left(\beta_1 X_1 + \dots + \beta_p X_p\right) \tag{13}$$

In our application we model two covariates: X_1 (0 for a good tracker, 1 for a poor tracker), and X_2 being the patient's total number of violations in the CPHM. The log rank test associated with the CPHM confirmed that the good tracker and poor tracker hazard rates, and the survival curves were significantly different (p-value = 0.0496), with the hazard rate for the poor trackers being 2.1 times that of good trackers, with a 95% confidence interval of [1.01, 4.38]. The associated hazard rate for poor trackers is shown to be 1.87 times that of good trackers, with a 95% confidence interval [0.75, 4.70]. By inclusion of the total number of second time violations the effect of tracking status has only reduced slightly, and it remains significant (1.87 versus 2.1).

4.2 Asseement of times to different violation counts and patient's last jump

Log-rank tests were likewise conducted to assess times to different violation counts. Let VX denote the violation times for the Xth violation and the DX's the associated event indicators (0 censored, 1 event of interest). Log rank tests for the two WPB tracking strata for selected violation times (X = 5, 10, 15, 20, 25, 30) showed significant differences between good and poor WPB trackers regarding the time to the patient's time to 10th violation (p = 0.027), their 15th (p = 0.025) and their 25th violation (p = 0.011). Likewise, significance at the 10% level was demonstrated for times to the patient's 5th, 20th and 30th violation (non-violatory lifetimes). All survival curves (not shown here) are significantly different or are close to being significant at the 5% level of significance. This confirms that the difference in time to violations between the good and poor trackers are consistently different, for these varying number of violations (VX, for X = 5, 10, 15, 20, 25, 30).

The time to a patient's last violation event was also investigated using log-rank tests and Kaplan–Meier curves. We examined nine levels of the effect of the following covariate, which categorises the counts the patient levels of violations as follows: 0–5 violations, 5–10, 10–15, 15–20, 20–25, 25–30, 30–40, 40–50 and >50 violations. A histogram of the time to a patient's last violation with boxplots of the times for each of these nine levels of categorisation shown is given in **Figure 20** (the number above the boxplots gives the number of patients in each of the nine categories).

Using the patient's time to their final violation/jump, as the event of interest, and implementing log-rank based tests using this covariate adjustment, the log rank test demonstrated a statistically significant difference between the survival curves of time to last violation (p-value <0.000001) across the above nine different total number of violation levels, {0–5, 5–10, 10–15, 15–20, 20–25, 25–30, 30–40, 40–50, >50 violations}.

Notably, the levels that most contribute to the difference between trackers and non-trackers are those patients who have a total number of violations between 10 and 15, between 20 and 25 and >50, in that order. A log rank test on time to last violation (time of last jump outside the WPB bands) as the outcome of interest by tracking

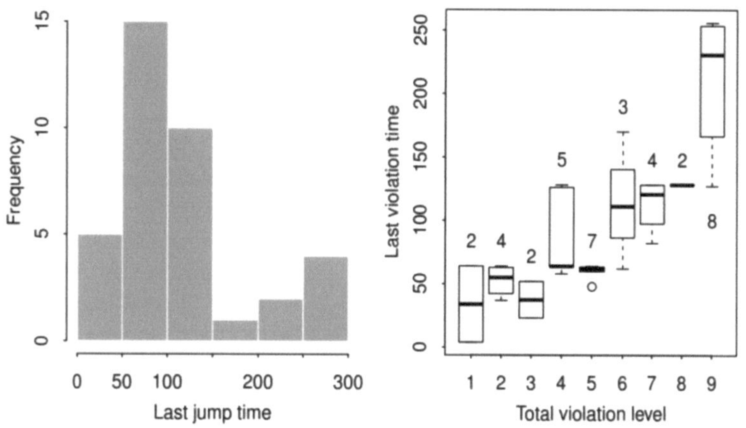

Figure 20.
Histogram and boxplots of time to last violation. The numbers above the boxplot (RHS) specify the number of patients in each violation level.

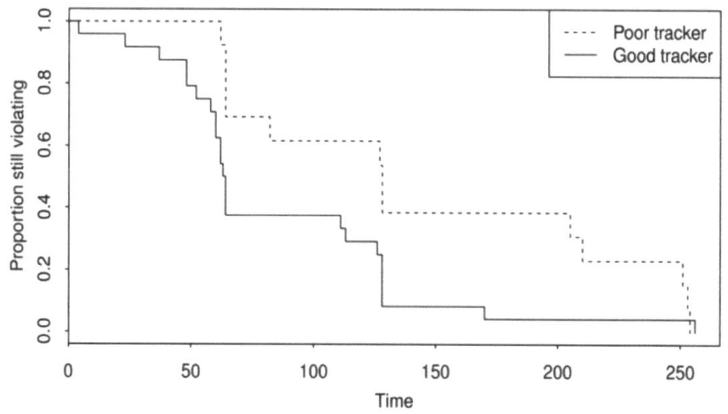

Figure 21.
Estimated survival curves for time to last violation by tracking status.

status, also establishes that there is a difference between the two survival curves (p-value = 0.045) (**Figure 21**). Clearly the WPB-based poor trackers tend to take longer to reach their last violation than good trackers. Corresponding Kaplan–Meier estimated curves are given in **Figure 21**. We note that up to ICU time 64 (≤64), 40% of the good versus 70% of the poor trackers are still violating, whereas after time point, 130, the corresponding percentages violating are 15% versus 40%, of the good versus poor trackers (**Figure 21**).

5. Conclusion

A log-rank test from the counting process formulation [37–39] established a significant difference between the hazard curves of the WPB-based good and poor trackers (p-value = 0.044). Similarly log-rank tests performed for a variety of violation numbers to test for differences between good and poor trackers times to their 5th, 10th, 15th, 20th, 25th and 30th violation, showed evidence of a significant difference between good and poor trackers for a selection of these violation times (namely patient's time to their 10th, 15th and 25th violation). In regard to analysing the patients time to their last recorded violation, log-rank tests and Kaplan–Meier curves showed that poor trackers tend to have a higher probability of still violating as time progresses in ICU compared to good trackers (p-value = 0.045).

Author details

Irene Hudson
Mathematical Sciences, School of Science, Royal Melbourne Institute of Technology, Melbourne, Victoria, Australia

*Address all correspondence to: irene.hudson@rmit.edu.au

References

[1] Nassar AP, Zampieri FG, Salluh JI, Bozza FA, Machado FR, Guimarães HP, et al. Organizational factors associated with target sedation on the first 48 h of mechanical ventilation: An analysis of checklist-ICU database. Critical Care (London, England). 2019;**23**(1):1-8. DOI: 10.1186/s13054-019-2323-y

[2] Sessler CN, Gosnell MS, Grap MJ, Brophy GM, O'Neal PV, Keane KA, et al. The Richmond Agitation-Sedation Scale: Validity and reliability in adult intensive care unit patients. American Journal of Respiratory and Critical Care Medicine. 2002;**166**(1):1338-1344. DOI: 10.1164/rccm.2107138

[3] Fraser GL, Riker RR. Monitoring sedation, agitation, analgesia, and delirium in critically ill adult patients. Critical Care Clinics. 2001;**17**(4):967-987. DOI: 10.1016/s0749-0704(05)70189-5

[4] Hochberg U, Sharon H, Bahir I, Brill S. Pain management - A decade's perspective of a new subspecialty. journal of pain. Research. 2021;**14**:923-930. DOI: 10.2147/JPR.S303815

[5] Pretorius A, Searle J, Marshall B. Barriers and enablers to emergency department nurses' management of patients' pain. Pain Management Nursing. 2015;**16**(3):372-379. DOI: 10.1016/j.pmn.2014.08.015

[6] Ucuzal M, Doğan R. Emergency nurses' knowledge, attitude and clinical decision making skills about pain. International Emergency Nursing. 2015;**23**(2):75-80. DOI: 0.1016/j.ienj.2014.11.006

[7] Varndell W, Fry M, Elliot D. Emergency nurses' perceptions of sedation management practices for critically ill intubated patients: A qualitative study. Journal of Clinical Nursing. 2015;**24**(21-22):3286-3295. DOI: 10.1111/jocn.12932

[8] Varndell W, Fry M, Elliot D. The validity, reliability, responsiveness and applicability of observation sedation-scoring instruments for use with adult patients in the emergency department: A systematic literature review. Australasian Emergency Nursing Journal. 2015;**18**(1):1-23. DOI: 10.1016/j.aenj.2014.07.001

[9] Kang I, Hudson IL, Rudge A, Chase JG. Wavelet Signatures and Diagnostics for the Assessment of ICU Agitation-Sedation Protocols. In: Olkkonen H, editor. Discrete Wavelet Transforms. 1st ed. Rijeka: IntechOpen; 2011. pp. 321-348. DOI: 10.5772/20547

[10] Kang I, Hudson IL, Rudge A, Chase JG. Density Estimation and Wavelet Thresholding via Bayesian Methods: A Wavelet Probability Band and Related Metrics Approach to Assess Agitation and Sedation in ICU Patients. In: Al-Asmari A, editor. Discrete Wavelet Transforms: A Compendium of New Approaches and Recent Applications. 1st ed. Rijeka: IntechOpen; 2013. pp. 127-162. DOI: 10.5772/52434. Available from: https://www.intechopen.com/chapters/42461

[11] Rudge AD, Chase JG, Shaw GM, Lee D, Wake GC, Hudson IL, et al. Impact of control on agitation-sedation dynamics. Control Engineering Practice. 2005;**13**(9):1139-1149. DOI: 10.1016/j.conengprac.2004.10.010

[12] Rudge AD, Chase JG, Shaw GM, Lee D. Physiological modelling of agitation-sedation dynamics including endogenous agitation reduction. Medical Engineering and Physics. 2006;**28**(7):629-638. DOI: 10.1016/j.medengphy.2005.10.008

[13] Rudge AD, Chase JG, Shaw GM, Lee D, Hann CE. Parameter identification and sedative sensitivity analysis of an agitation-sedation model. Computer Methods and Programs in Biomedicine. 2006;**83**(3):211-221. DOI: 10.1016/j.cmpb.2006.06.011

[14] Chase JG, Rudge AD, Shaw GM, Wake GC, Lee D, Hudson IL. Modeling and control of the agitation-sedation cycle for critical care patients. Medical Engineering and Physics. 2004;**26**(6): 459-471. DOI: 10.1016/j.medengphy. 2004.02.001

[15] Olson DWM, Zomorodi MG, James ML, Cox CE, Moretti EW, Riemen KE, et al. Exploring the impact of augmenting sedation assessment with physiologic monitors. Australian Critical Care. 2014;**27**(3):145-150. DOI: 10.1016/ J.AUCC.2013.09.001

[16] Barbato M, Barclay G, Potter J, Yeo W, Chung J. Correlation between observational scales of sedation and comfort and bispectral index scores. Journal of Pain and Symptom Management. 2017;**54**:186-193

[17] West N, McBeth PB, Brodie SM, van Heusden K, Sunderland S, Ga D, et al. Feasibility of continuous sedation monitoring in critically ill intensive care unit patients using the NeuroSENSE WAV $_{\text{CNS}}$ index. Journal of Clinical Monitoring and Computing. 2018;**32**(6):1081-1091. DOI: 10.1007/s10877-018-0115-6

[18] Milane TA, Bennett ED, Grounds RM. Isoflurane and propofol for long-term sedation in the intensive care unit. A crossover study. Anaesthesia. 1992;**47**(9):768-774. DOI: 10.1111/ j.1365-2044.1992.tb03254.x

[19] Barr J, Fraser FL, Puntillo K, Ely GC, Dasta EW, Davidson JE, et al. Clinical practice guidelines for the management of pain, agitation, and delirium in adult patients in the intensive care unit. Critical Care Medicine. 2013;**41**(1):263-306. DOI: 10.1097/CCM.0b013e3182783b72

[20] Vincent J, Shehabi Y, Walsh TS, Pandharipande PP, Ball JA, Spronk P, et al. Intensive Care Medicine. 2016; **42**(6):962-971. DOI: 10.1007/ s00134-016-4297-4

[21] Kress JP, Pohlman AS, Hall JB. Sedation and analgesia in the intensive care unit. American Journal of Respiratory and Critical Care Medicine. 2002;**166**(8): 1024-1028. DOI: 10.1164/ rccm.200204-270CC

[22] Allignol A, Schumacher M, Beyersmann J. Empirical transition matrix of multi-state models: The etm package. Journal of Statistical Software. 2011;**38**(4): 1-14. DOI: 10.18637/jss.v038.i04

[23] Nießl A, Allignol A, Beyersmann J, Mueller C. Statistical inference for state occupation and transition probabilities in non-Markov multi-state models subject to both random left-truncation and right-censoring. Econometrics and Statistics. 2021. ISSN 2452-3062. Available from: https://www.sciencedirect.com/science/ article/pii/S2452306221001155

[24] Andersen PK, Borgan O, Gill RD, Keiding N. Statistical Models Based on Counting Processes. 3rd ed. Vol. 784. New York: Springer; 2012. DOI: 10.1007/ 978-1-4612-4348-9

[25] Commenges D, Barberfer-Gateau P, Dartigues JF, Loiseau P, Salamon R. A non-homogeneous markov chain model for follow-up studies with application to epilepsy. Methods of Information Medicine. 1984;**23**(2):109-114. DOI: 10.1007/s00239-009-9282-x

[26] Snappin SM, Jiang Q, Iglewicz B. Illustrating impact of a Time-varying

covariate with an extended Kaplan-Meier Estimator. Amer. Statist. 2005; **59**(4):301-307. DOI: 10.1198/000313005X70371

[27] Hudson IL, Tursunalieva AT. Copula thresholds and modelling Agitation-Sedation (A-S) in ICU: Analysis of nurses scores of A-S and automated drug infusions by protocol. InTechOpen. 2022 (to appear)

[28] Tursunalieva, A., Hudson, I., Chase, J. Copula modelling of nurses' agitation-sedation rating of ICU patients, in Communications in Computer and Information Science 1150: SDS, 2019. Simone Diniz Junqueira Barbosa, et al (ed.), Springer Nature Singapore Pte Ltd. H. Nguyen (Ed.): RSSDS 2019, CCIS 1150, 148–161, 2019. DOI: 10.1007/978-981-15-1960-4_11

[29] Tursunalieva, A. Hudson, I., Chase, J. 2019, 'Copula modelling of nurses' agitation-sedation rating of ICU patients: towards monitoring and health alerting tools', in Proceedings from the 23rd International Congress on Modelling and Simulation, Sondoss Elsawah (ed.), Modelling & Simulation Society of Australia & New Zealand (MSSANZ), Melbourne, Australia, pp. 835-841. ISBN: 978-0-9758400-9-2. Available from: https://mssanz.org.au/modsim2019/I4/tursunalieva.pdf

[30] Aalen OO, Borgan Ø, Gjessing HK. Survival and Event History Analysis: A Process Point of View. 1st ed. New York: Springer; 2008. p. 560. DOI 10.1007/978-0-387-68560-1

[31] Aalen O, Johansen S. An empirical transition matrix for non-homogeneous Markov chains based on censored observations. Scandinavian Journal of Statistics. 1978;**5**(3):141-150. Available from: https://www.jstor.org/stable/4615704

[32] Beyersmann J, Wolkewitz M, Allignol A, Grambauer N, Schumacher M. Application of multistate models in hospital epidemiology: advances and challenges. Biometrical Journal. 2011;**53**:332-350. DOI: 10.1002/bimj.201000146

[33] Munoz-Price LS, Frencken FJ, Tarima S, Bonten M. Handling time dependent variables: Antibiotics and antibiotic resistance. Clinical Infectious Diseases. 2016;**62**(12):1558-1563. DOI: 10.1093/cid/ciw191

[34] Andersen P, Keiding N. Multi-state models for event history analysis. Statistical Methods in Medical Research. 2002;**11**(2):91-115. DOI: 10.1191/0962280202SM276ra

[35] Commenges D. Multi-state models in epidemiology. Lifetime Data Analysis. 1999;**5**(4):315-327. DOI: 10.1023/a:1009636125294

[36] Commenges D. Inference for multi-state models from interval-censored data. Statistical Methods in Medical Research. 2002;**11**(2):167-182. DOI: 10.1191/0962280202sm279ra

[37] Simon R, Makuch R. A non-parametric graphical representation of the relationship between survival and the occurrence of an event: application to re- sponder versus non-responder bias. Statistics in Medicine. 1984;**3**:35-44. DOI: 10.1002/sim.4780030106

[38] Broström G. Event History Analysis with R. ISBN: Chapman and Hall/CRC; 2022. p. 9781138587717

[39] Broström G. Event History Analysis with R. 2nd ed. Boca Raton: Chapman & Hall/CRC; 2012. 236p. Available from: https://www.routledge.com/Event-History-Analysis-with-R/Brostrom/p/book/9781138587717

Chapter 4

Copula Modelling of Agitation-Sedation (A-S) in ICU: Threshold Analysis of Nurses' Scores of A-S and Automated Drug Infusions by Protocol

Irene Hudson, Ainura Tursunalieva and J. Geoffrey Chase

Abstract

Pain management is increasingly recognised as a formal medical subspecialty worldwide. Empirical distributions of the nurses' ratings of a patient's pain and/or agitation levels and the administered dose of sedative are often positively skewed, and if the joint distribution is non-elliptical, then high nurses' ratings of a patient's agitation levels may not correspond to the true occurrences of patient's agitation-sedation (A-S). Copulas are used to capture such nonlinear dependence between skewed distributions and check for the presence of lower (LT) and/or upper tail (UT) dependence between the nurses' A-S rating and the automated sedation dose, thus finding thresholds and regions of mismatch between the nurse's scores and automated sedation dose, thereby suggesting a possible way forward for an improved alerting system for over- or under-sedation. We find for LT dependence nurses tend to underestimate the patient's agitation in the moderate agitation zone. In the mild agitation zone, nurses tend to assign a rating, that is, on average, 0.30 to 0.45 points lower than expected for the patient's given agitation severity. For UT dependence in the moderate agitation zone, nurses tend to either moderately or strongly underestimate patient's agitation, but in periods of severe agitation, nurses tend to overestimate a patient's agitation. Our approach lends credence to augmenting conventional RASS and SAS agitation measures with semi-automated systems and identifying thresholds and regions of deviance for alerting increased risk.

Keywords: copula dependence, K-plots, agitation-sedation (A-S) control, thresholds, nurses' scores

1. Introduction

Pain management is becoming increasingly recognised as a formal medical subspecialty worldwide. Pain is the most common reason that patients come to the emergency department. Emergency nurses have an indispensable role in the management of this pain [1]. Sedation in the intensive care unit (ICU) is challenging, as both over- and under-sedation are detrimental [2]. Optimal sedation and analgesic strategies, combined with delirium management, are difficult when caring for critically ill patients. For sedation monitoring, the most widely used tools are the Richmond Agitation and Sedation Scale (RASS) [3] and Sedation Agitation Scale (SAS) [4]. Assessments using RASS and SAS are undertaken intermittently and traditionally rely on patients' behavioural response to stimulation, which perturbs rest and sleep [5–8]. Various studies have suggested that a non-stimulating method for "continuous" sedation monitoring may be beneficial and allow for more frequent assessment.

Indeed earlier, Rudge, Chase, and Shaw [9] discussed target-controlled infusion (TCI) systems to deliver drugs to maintain target plasma concentrations, using a pharmacokinetic model, shown to be feasible when anaesthesia is given over short periods of reduced consciousness and well-known pharmacology is invoked. Infusion systems that regulate the infusion rate to maintain target agitation levels, to regulate the primary metric for long-term sedation, are one approach to improving care in the ICU. The data analysed in this chapter pertains to the scenario and data type studied earlier by Hudson, Rudge and colleagues [9–14].

These authors have suggested that assessing the severity of agitation is a challenging clinical problem as variability related to drug metabolism for each individual is often subjective. A multitude of previous studies also suggest assessment accuracy of the sedation quality conducted by nurses tend to suffer from subjectivity and lead to sub-optimal sedation [9–14]. For example, it has been recommended by some authors to use lighter than deeper levels of sedation. And that sedation should be reviewed and adjusted regularly [5–8]. Agitation management methods frequently rely on subjective agitation assessment the carers then select an appropriate infusion rate based upon their evaluation of these scales, experience, and intuition [3–5]. This approach usually leads to largely continuous infusions which lack a bolus-focused approach, commonly resulting in over or under-sedation.

The work of [9–14] aimed to enhance feedback protocols for medical decision support systems and eventually automated sedation administration. A minimal differential equation model to predict or simulate each patient's agitation-sedation status over time was presented in [9] for our ICU patients and was shown to capture patient agitation-sedation (A-S) dynamics. The use of quantitative modelling to enhance understanding of the agitation-sedation (A-S) system and the provision of an A-S simulation platform is one of the key tools in this area of patient critical care. A more refined A-S model, which utilised regression with an Epanechnikov kernel was formulated by [9]. A Bayesian approach using densities and wavelet shrinkage methods was later suggested by [10] to assess a previously derived deterministic, parametric A-S model [11], thus successfully challenging the practice of sedating ICU patients using continuous infusions.

Wavelets approaches [10, 11] were shown to provide reliable diagnostics and visualisation tools to assess A-S models, giving alternative metrics of A-S control to assess the validity of the earlier A-S deterministic models (**Table 3** in [10]). This suite of wavelet metrics based on the discrete wavelet transform (DWT) established the value of earlier deterministic agitation-sedation (A-S) models against empirical (recorded) dynamic A-S infusion profiles, providing robust performance metrics of A-S control and excellent tools, based on the classification of patients into poor and good trackers based on Wavelet Probability Bands (WPBs). Importantly, the WPBs were shown to be a useful patient-specific method by which to identify and detect regions in the patient's A-S profile i.e., times whilst in ICU, where the simulated infusion rate performs poorly, thus providing visual and quantified ways to help improve and distil the deterministic A-S model and in practice be a gauge to alert carers.

The aim of this chapter is to identify regions of poor and good control using copulas. Copulas are functions that join or connect multivariate distribution functions to their one-dimensional marginal distribution functions. Copulas have had applications in fields such as finance [15, 16], public health and medicine [17], and actuarial science [18, 19]. Empirical distributions of the nurses' ratings of a patient's pain and/or agitation levels and the administered dose of sedative are often positively skewed and if the joint distribution is non-elliptical, then high nurses' ratings of a patient's agitation levels may not correspond to the occurrences of patient's A-S profile with large infusion dose. Copulas are used as they measure nonlinear dependencies capturing the dependence between skewed distributions. Copulas are widely applied in diverse fields, including health services research and medical studies, quantitative risk management, econometric modelling, environmental studies, finance, and hydrology.

Advantages of using copulas in modelling are: (i) capacity to model both linear and non-linear dependence; (ii) allowing an arbitrary choice of a marginal distribution; and (iii) capability of modelling extreme endpoints. Copulas are functions that "couple together" the marginal cumulative distribution functions (CDFs) of a random vector to form its joint CDF. When used in statistical modelling, copulas can estimate multivariate distributions of data involving two or more outcome variables for mixed type, complex data. We determine the best-fit copula type for all patients with a focus on differences between poor and good trackers, where classification of patients into poor and good trackers was based on Wavelet Probability Bands (WPB) [10, 11].

This chapter builds on the earlier pilot work of Tursunalieva et al. [20, 21]] to address the gap in the methodology by integrating non-elliptical dependence structure between nurses' rating of a patient's agitation level and the automated sedation dose. In an earlier pilot work discussed by Hudson [22], the tail thresholds of two (2) test patients were determined manually, whereas in [21] the dynamic programming algorithm of Bai and Perron [23] was used to establish the lower and upper tail threshold. Copula mathematics allows us to determine and identify lower and/or upper tail thresholds when they exist for all 36 intensive care unit patients' agitation-sedation profiles collected at Christchurch Hospital, School of Medicine and Health Sciences, NZ and analysed earlier in [9–14]. Infusion data were recorded using an electronic drug infusion device for all admitted ICU patients during a nine-month observation period and required more than 24 hours of sedation.

In this chapter, our novel and general formulation of the equation relating each patient's nurses' score to the automated infusion dose is given by the following expression nurses' score = intercept+α*Dose–β*Dose*LT region+ γ*Dose*UT region. This formulation accounts for the non-linear relationships between the nurses' A-S rating and the automated sedation dose, and permits identification of thresholds and regions of mismatch between the nurse's scores and sedation dose, thereby suggesting a possible way forward for an improved alerting system for over/under-sedation.

Establishing the presence of tail dependence and patient-specific thresholds for areas with different agitation intensities has significant implications for the effective administration of sedatives. Better management of A-S states will allow clinicians to improve the efficacy of care and reduce healthcare costs. Our approach lends credence to augmenting conventional RASS and SAS agitation measures with semi-automated systems [24–26] and identifying thresholds and regions of deviance for alerting increased risk. Better management of A-S states will allow clinicians to improve the efficacy of care and reduce healthcare costs.

1.1 Data and methods

This chapter models the agitation-sedation profiles of 36 patients collected at the Christchurch Hospital, Christchurch School of Medicine and Health Sciences, NZ. Two measures were recorded for each patient: (1) the nurses' ratings/scores of a patient's agitation level, and (2) an automated sedation dose (see **Figure 1**). Infusion data were recorded using an electronic drug infusion device for all admitted ICU patients during a nine-month observation period and required more than 24 hours of sedation. Infusion data containing less than 48 hours of continuous data, or data from patients whose sedation requirements were extreme, such as those with severe head injuries, were excluded [9, 10].

A total of 36 ICU patients met these requirements and were enrolled in the study. Classification of patients into poor and good trackers, based on the Wavelet Probability Bands (WPB), is given in **Table 1**. The so-called good tracker delineates the scenario where the nurse's rating scores remains within the (time-based) 90% coverage of wavelet probability band (WPB) based on the simulated dose profiles [10, 11]. Poor tracking delineates the scenario where the nurses' rating scores remain outside the (time based) 90% coverage of wavelet probability band (WPB) for a significant portion of time based on the simulated dose profiles [11].

By way of illustration, we carefully examine four patients from the pool of 36 patients. **Tables 2** and **3** summarise each of these 4 patients' WPB tracker status, time to first, second and third violation outside the WPB bands, their total number of violations over ICU stay, and patient's time in ICU, along with their specific WPB% value. Display of their line profiles of *nurses' rating* of A-S in relation to drug infusion *dose* over time, for each of the 4 patients (P8, P27, P18, P28) are given in **Figures 2–4**.

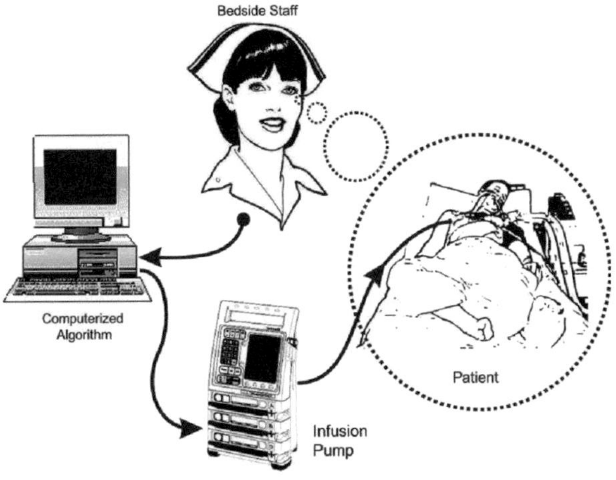

Figure 1.
Diagram of the feedback loop employing nursing staff's feedback of subjectively assessed patient agitation through the infusion controller (diagram is sourced from Chase et al.) [12, 14].

WPB [11]	WCORR [10]	Chase et al. [14]	Rudge et al. [9]
2	2	—	—
4	4	—	—
—	—	6	—
7	7	7	7
10	10	—	10
11	11	—	11
—	—	12	—
—	—	—	13
—	—	17	—
21	21	21	—
22	22	—	22
27	27	27	27
28	28	—	28
—	29	—	29
32	32	—	—
33	33	—	33
34	34	34	—
—	35	—	35
Total: N_1 = 12	**Total: N_2 = 14**	**Total: N_3 = 7**	**Total: N_4 = 10**

Low WPB 90% values under 70% indicate a poor tracker by Kang's WPB diagnostics [11].

Table 1.
Patient numbers of the **poor** *trackers according to the criteria of 4 studies, developed earlier in [11].*

	V1	V2	V3	Total V's	Time in ICU	WPB%
P8/Good	1	2	3	46	128	87.5%
P27/Poor	1	4	5	89	225	43.7%

Table 2.
Time to the patient-specific, 1st violation denoted by V1, second violation V2 and third violation V3, total number of violations, total ICU time and WPB% values.

	V1	V2	V3	Total V's	Time in ICU	WPB%
P18/Good	2	24	26	20	64	93.8%
P28/Poor	1	5	12	114	203	50.8%

Tablc 3.
Time to the patient-specific, 1st violation V1, second violation V2, and third violation V3, total number of violations, total ICU time and WPB% values.

Note that a violation event occurs when the nurses observed agitation score or rating is outside either the lower or upper limits of the 90%WPB bands associated with the patient's automated infusion dose trajectory over time in ICU.

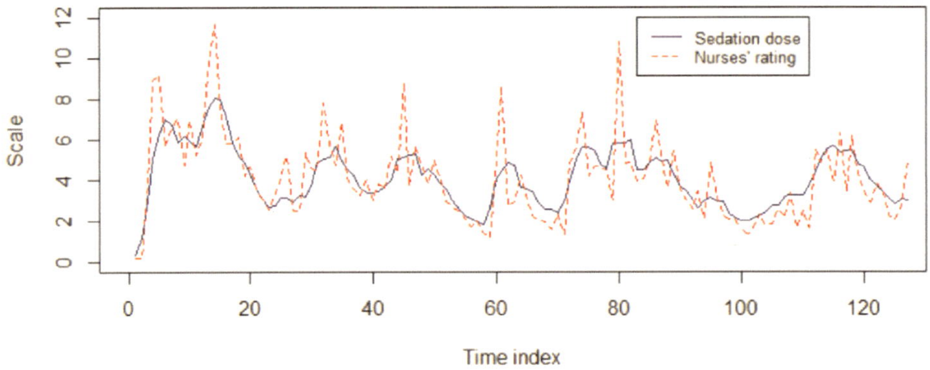

Figure 2.
Line plot of nurses' rating of patient agitation and the automated sedation dose for patient 8 (WPB-based good tracker).

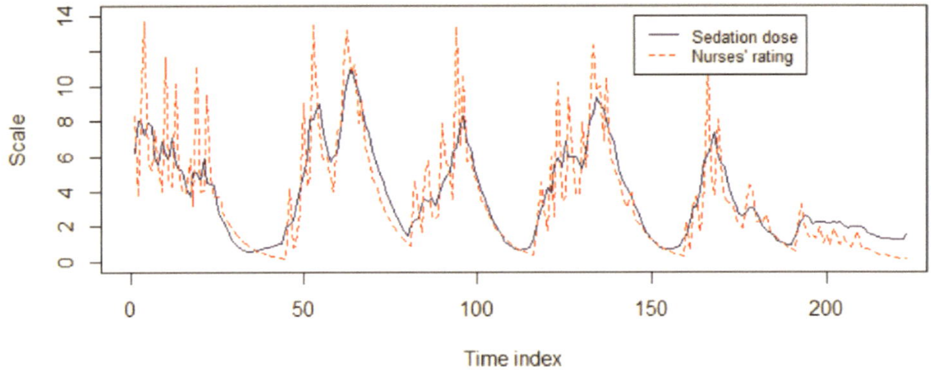

Figure 3.
Line plot of nurses' rating of patient agitation and the automated sedation dose for patient 27 (WPB-based poor tracker).

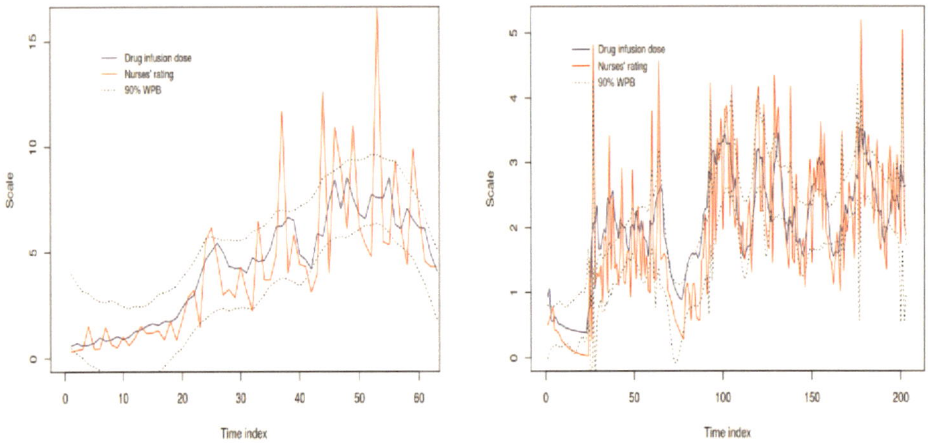

Figure 4.
Line plot (WPB% bands), patient 18 (LHS, good) and 28 (RHS, poor tracker).

The first patient (patient 8) in **Table 2** is a good WPB tracker and the second (patient 27) a poor WPB tracker both studied in [20, 21], for which the upper tail thresholds of the nurses' scores using copulas were established, in a pilot study of these 2 patients using copula mathematics. We also refer the reader to Hudson's chapter in this book "Modelling Agitation-Sedation (A-S) in ICU: an Empirical Transition and Time to event analysis of poor and good tracking between nurses scores and automated A-S measures" [22].

The corresponding WPB% values for patient 8 and patient 27 are 87.5% and 43.7%, respectively (**Table 2**). Overall, the minimum, median and maximum WPB % values for the 24 good trackers is (58.8%, 87.5%, 96.9%) and (47.3%, 64.8%, 77.3%) for the 12 poor trackers (**Table 1**). Noteworthy also is that the A-S time series of these two patients examined (P8 and P27) were of disparate lengths - patient 8 had 10,561 time points and patient 27, had 13,441 time points. The full set of patients studied had a range of [3001-25,261] time points of automated dose assessments.

Patient 18 (good tracker) with a WPB% of 93.8% and patient 28 (poor tracker) with WPB% of 50.8% (**Table 3**) were studied in detail in [20, 21], for which both upper and lower tails/thresholds of over or under-estimation of agitation levels by the nurses' rating were established using copula dependence analytics (see also [27–29]).

Patients vary according to their length of stay in ICU and consequently differ in their opportunity for violations to occur. The good trackers generally have shorter ICU time and thus less chance to exhibit an increased total number of violations.

The total number of WPB-based violations is greater for the poor trackers than for the good trackers, and it is the poor trackers that tend to have longer ICU times. There are three approximate categories of patient ICU time: 50−64, 113−128, and 205–256, and 19 of the 36 patients have an ICU time of $\leq$64.

2. Methodology

2.1 Copula formulation

In our study, the copula models aim to capture the dependence between the observed/recorded nurses' rating and the automated sedation dose for each patient. We test for and utilise the so-called best fitting copula found. This section acts as a guide to decide if there exists a tail relationship between the nurses' rating of patient agitation A-S score and automated sedation dose.

Analytically and contextually, the lower tail region corresponds to the patient specific *mild agitation range* and the upper tail region corresponds to the *severe agitation range*, with the non-tail middle region capturing the patient's *moderate agitation range*. Clearly patient's transition between these so-called mild, moderate and severe ranges or states over time in ICU. In our context, if the two distributions that is of nurses' (observed) rating and that of the automated sedation dose are independent univariate Gaussians, then we can define the multivariate Gaussian distribution as the best fit. Let X and Y be independent Gaussian (with arbitrary means and variances), then $Z_j = a_{j1}X + a_{j2}Y$ is univariate Gaussian for j = 1, 2, ... , n and a_{j1}, a_{j2} are real constants, and Z is multivariate Gaussian.

Let $Z = \begin{pmatrix} Z_1 \\ \vdots \\ Z_n \end{pmatrix} = A \begin{pmatrix} X \\ Y \end{pmatrix}$ be constructed based on the $n \times n$ matrix A where X and Y.

are independent and identically distributed (i.i.d.) N(0,1) random variables. Then $Z + \mu$ is multivariate Gaussian with mean vector μ and covariance matrix $= AA^T$. From the Central Limit Theorem, the Gaussian distribution arises as a limit of a scaled sum of weakly dependent random variables [27, 28].

Parametric copula families are conventionally constructed to satisfy different combinations of bivariate dependence structures with tail behaviours [28]. The general definition of Archimedean copulas is given by Boateng [29]. It is noteworthy that the Clayton, Gumbel, and Frank copulas are examples of existing Archimedean copulas. A discussion about the Clayton, Gumbel, and Frank copulas, and tail dependence of a bivariate copula, Kendall's tau representations, and copula models of the Clayton, Frank, and Gumbel copulas are also defined in [29]. The Clayton copula, for example, accommodates only lower tail dependence [30], the Frank copula allows dependence around the mode [31], and the Gumbel is relevant only when upper tail dependence exists [32]. The difference between the Clayton and Gumbel copulas is: (i) for the Clayton copula, correlations on the extreme left sides of distributions are more concentrated (i.e., higher correlations) than those in the extreme right sides of the distributions, and (ii) for the Gumbel copula, the correlations on the extreme right sides of distributions are more concentrated (i.e., higher correlations) than those in the extreme left sides of the distributions. The visuals in Section 3 of this chapter illustrate these trends. We refer the reader to Boeting [29] and below give the bivariate Gaussian formulation and bivariate Frank and Gumbel copula, as three examples.

Bivariate Gaussian copula

The copula cdf is:

$$C(u, v, \rho) = \Phi_2\left(\Phi^{-1}(u), \Phi^{-1}(v); \rho\right), 0 < u, v < 1. \tag{1}$$

Bivariate Frank

For $-\infty < \delta < \infty$, the copula cdf is:

$$C(u, v, \delta) = -\delta^{-1} log \left(\frac{1 - e^{-\delta} - \left(1 - e^{-\delta u}\right)\left(1 - e^{-\delta v}\right)}{1 - e^{-\delta}} \right), 0 < u, v < 1. \tag{2}$$

Bivariate Gumbel copula

The copula cdf is: $C(u, v, \delta) = exp\left\{ -\left([-\log u]^{\delta} + [-\log v]^{\delta} \right)^{1/\delta} \right\}$, $0 \le u, v \le 1, 1 \le \delta \le \infty$. Upper tail dependence function for Gumbel copula is:

$$b_U(w_1 w_2; \delta) = w_1 + w_2 - \left(w_1^{\delta} + w_2^{\delta}\right)^{1/\delta}. \tag{3}$$

2.2 Kendall K-plot construction

The best fitting copula was selected by maximum likelihood estimation, except for the t-copula, for which the degrees of freedom parameter is found by a crude profile likelihood optimisation over the interval (2, 10]. We use the Kendall plot

(K-plot) [33] to determine the bivariate patient-specific thresholds in the cases where the best fitting copula has tails. The K-plot splits the data into two regions with significantly different strengths of dependence between nurses' rating and the automated sedation dose, namely: (1) the main region with an approximately linear relationship; and (2) the tail regions with a non-linear relationship. Recently the K-plot has gained popularity with regard to its association with the receiver operating characteristic (ROC) curve, a pivotal biostatistical graphical tool traditionally used for testing the ability of biomarkers to discriminate between populations [34].

The K-plot adopts the familiar probability plot (Q-Q plot) to detect dependence. A lack of linearity of the standard Q-Q plot is an indication of non-normality of the distribution of a random variable. Similarly, in the absence of association between two variables, the K-plot is close to a straight line, while the amount of curvature in the K-plot is characteristic of the degree of dependence in the data, and is related, in a definite way, to the underlying copula. This method is closely related to Kendall's tau statistic [35] from which it takes the name. For more details refer to [27, 33].

To construct a K-plot, we need to compute H_i defined for a given pair (X_i, Y_i) with $1 \le i \le n$ as follows: $H_i = \#\{j \ne i : X_j \le X_i, Y_j \le Y_i\}/(n-1)$. Next, we need to order the variable H_i, $H_{(1)} \le \ldots \le H_{(n)}$ and plot the pairs $\left(W_{1:n}, H_{(i)}\right), 1 \le i \le n$, where W_(1,n) is the expectation of the ith order statistic in a random sample of size n from the distribution K_0 of the H_i under the null hypothesis of independence. Using the definition of the density of an order statistic, we define the form of K_0 under the null hypothesis of the independence, as follows:

$$W_{1:n} = n\binom{n-1}{i-1}\int_0^1 \omega\{K_0(\omega)\}^{i-1} \times \{1 - K_0(\omega)\}^{n-1} dK_0(\omega), 1 \le i \le n. \tag{4}$$

2.3 Multiple threshold identification via dynamic programming algorithm

To identify a patient-specific threshold, we apply the dynamic programming algorithm discussed in Section 3.3 of [23] to use the dependence measure H_i. This algorithm captures multiple thresholds; however, to be consistent with the objective of this paper, we focus on determining the lower and upper tail thresholds. In our study, the lower tail threshold corresponds to the lowest (lower) threshold and the upper tail threshold corresponds to the highest (upper) threshold, respectively for either dose or the nurses' score profiles.

2.4 Prediction equation of nurses' score with respect to dose allowing for tails

Below we detail, as an illustration to the novel method that accommodates lower and upper thresholds beyond conventional correlational analysis using Kendall tau and copulas, the resultant equations specific to two patients, Patient 20 and Patient 8, which are both good trackers. P20 has no tails and P8 a lower tail. All the patients' equations and their details are tabulated in the Appendix A.

The general formulation of the equation relating each patient's nurses' score to the automated infusion dose is given by either of the following expressions:

- Score = intercept + α* Dose–β Dose * LT + γ Dose * UT

- $\text{Score} = \text{intercept} + \text{slope(Dose)}–(\text{slope} : \text{Lower region})\ \text{Dose} + (\text{slope dose} : \text{Upper region}).$

Patient 20: The recorded or so-called nurses' observed A-S score and the automated sedation dose for patient 20 are independent univariate Gaussians, therefore, their joint distribution is Gaussian (**Tables 4** and **5** and LHS of **Figure 5**). This gives a bivariate Gaussian copula, with neither lower nor upper tails (RHS of **Figure 5**). Thus, the relationship between P20's nurses' score and infusion dose is estimated using a simple linear regression (SLR) equation, score = intercept + α*dose, with intercept and slope parameters − 0.31 and α = 1.16, respectively (**Table 6** and RHS of **Figure 5**).

Patient 8: In contrast to patient 20, for patient 8 (good tracker) the nurses' recorded score and the automated sedation dose are skewed distributions (**Figure 6**), with the joint distribution being Survival Gumbel with a lower tail dependence. (lower tail *tau* = 0.70)

Patient 20 – good, no tails	Estimate	Standard Error	t value	P value	
Intercept	−0.311	0.22	−1.41	0.16	NS
Dose	1.156	0.104	11.06	<2e-16	***
*Adjusted R-squared: 0.49, Signif. codes: 0 '***' 0.001 '**' 0.01 '*' 0.05 '.' 0.1 ' ' 1.*					

Table 4.
Patient 20 equation components and p-values, good tracker, no tails.

Patient 8 - good, lower tail	Estimate	Standard Error	t value	P value	
Dose	1.012	0.0848	14.3	<2e-16	***
Dose*LT	−0.2849	0.0966	−2.95	0.0045	**
*Adjusted R-squared: 0.766, Signif. codes: 0 '***' 0.001 '**' 0.01 '*' 0.05 '.' 0.1 ' ' 1.*					

Table 5.
Patient 8 (P8) equation components - good tracker, lower tail tau = 0.70.

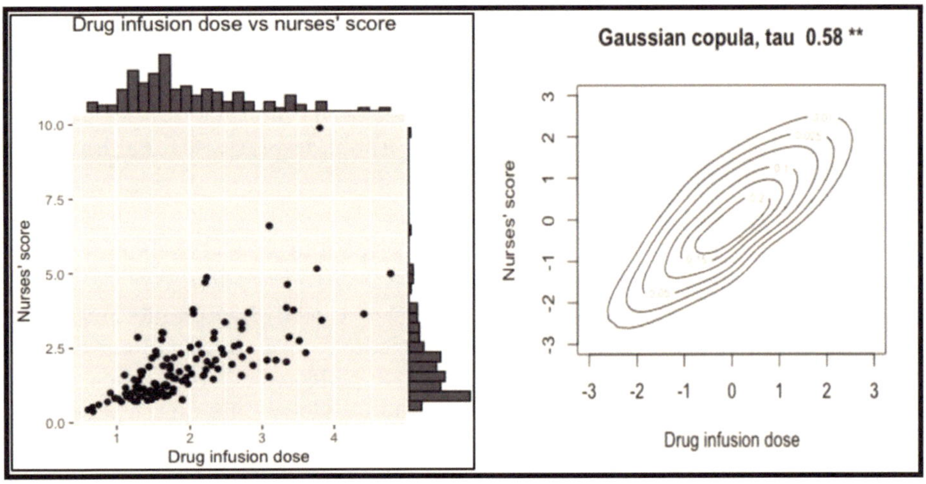

Figure 5.
Bivariate plots (LHS), copula type, and relevant tau (RHS) relating P 20's nurses' A-S score with dose, good tracker, no tails. SLR line is not shown.

Copula types	Tail	No. of copulas	WPB good trackers (Patient no.)	WPB poor trackers (Patient no.)
Clayton	Lower	2	P3, P19	
Rotated Tawn type 1, 180 degrees	Lower	1		**P35**
Survival Gumbel	Lower	7	P1, P5, P6, P8, P14	**P2**, P7
Survival Joe	Lower	2	**P15**	**P28**
BB8	No tails	2	P30, P36	
Frank	No tails	5	P13	P10, P11, **P27**, P33
Gaussian	No tails	5	P12, P17, P20, P29	P21
Survival BB8	No tails	7	P16, P18, P24, P26, P31	P22, P34
Survival BB7	Two tails	1		**P32**
t copula	Two Tails	1	**P25**	
Gumbel	Upper	2	**P23**	**P4**
Joe	Upper	1	**P37**	

Table 6.
List of copulas selected as optimal for the 36 patients (13 poor trackers). Shaded rows indicate the poor trackers. PX denotes patient number X.

(see **Table 7** and **Figure 6**, top panel). Hence, the relationship between P8's nurses' score and the dose is estimated by our novel prediction equation, as follows.

Score = 1.01Dose-0.29Dose*LT: The corresponding slope and lower tail parameters are $\alpha = 1.01$ and $\beta = -0.29$ (**Table 7**). The highly significant slope of 1.01 ($p < 0.00001$) indicates that in this patient's moderate agitation zone nurses tend to estimate agitation severity quite accurately. However, in the mild agitation zone, nurses tend to assign a rating that is, on average, 0.29 points lower than expected for the patient's given (by automated dose) agitation severity ($p = 0.0045$) (RHS of bottom panel of **Figure 6**). There are 33 (out of a total of 127) such occurrences indicating that in approximately one in every four ratings, nurses tend to underestimate this patients' agitation severity, LT dose threshold = 3.02 and LT score threshold = 2.57.

The Kendall-plot is then used to identify the lower tail threshold which occurs at the 26th percentile in the patient's bivariate (dose, score) trajectory (**Table A.1** Appendix), estimated by the algorithm of Bai and Perron [23]. For patient 8, the LT infusion dose threshold is 3.02 and LT nurse's score threshold is 2.57 (see percentiles in **Table A.1**) and the full set of equations in **Table A.2** in Appendix.

3. Results

3.1 Copula types across WPB status and tails status, and copula *taus*

Table 4 Gives the summary of copulas distributions selected as optimal for the total 36 patients stratified by WPB tracking status, copula type, number and type of tail(s), as gleaned from the more detailed **Table 5**, which gives each patient's WPB status, number of time points captured over ICU stay, patient's copula type, in

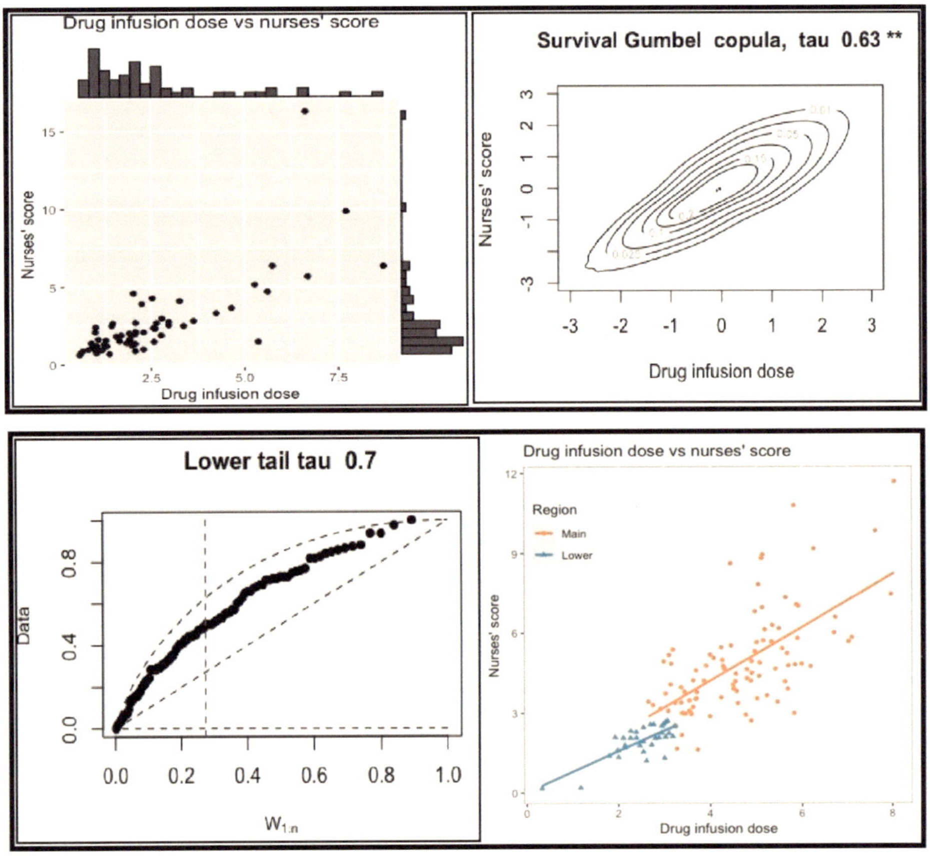

Figure 6.
P8 bivariate plots (LHS), copula type and main region tau (upper panel) and K-plot and lower tail (LT) tau = 0.70, with fit lines (bottom panel) relating P8's score with dose. P8 is a good tracker with lower tail thresholds for dose and nurses' score: LT dose threshold = 3.02 and LT nurses' score threshold = 2.57.

Patient no.	WPB status	Time			Copula tau (τ)		
		n	Copula type	Tail	Main region	Lower tail	Upper tail
1		59	Survival Gumbel	Lower	0.56	0.67	
2	Poor	63	Survival Gumbel	Lower	0.53	0.64	
3		63	Clayton	Lower	0.49	0.66	
4	Poor	63	Gumbel	**Upper**	0.61		0.69
5		48	Survival Gumbel	Lower	0.44	0.55	
6		63	Survival Gumbel	Lower	0.48	0.57	
7	Poor	63	Survival Gumbel	Lower	0.82	0.85	
8		127	Survival Gumbel	Lower	0.63	0.70	
10	Poor	255	Frank		0.67		
11	Poor	111	Frank		0.71		
12		127	Gaussian		0.56		
13		63	Frank		0.74		

Patient no.	WPB status	Time			Copula tau (τ)		
		n	Copula type	Tail	Main region	Lower tail	Upper tail
14		49	Survival Gumbel	Lower	0.65	0.72	
15		63	Survival Joe	Lower	0.53	0.74	
16		127	Survival BB8		0.67		
17		63	Gaussian		0.52		
18		63	Survival BB8		0.69		
19		127	Clayton	Lower	0.54	0.69	
20		127	Gaussian		0.58		
21	Poor	61	Gaussian		0.57		
22	Poor	127	Survival BB8		0.64		
23		57	Gumbel	**Upper**	0.61		0.68
24		127	Survival BB8		0.64		
25		**63**	**t copula**	**Both**	**0.57**	**0.06**	**0.06**
26		63	Survival BB8		0.64		
27	Poor	223	Frank		0.70		
28	Poor	203	Survival Joe	Lower	0.59	0.79	
29		53	Gaussian		0.68		
30		60	BB8		0.46		
31		255	Survival BB8		0.68		
32	**Poor**	**252**	Survival BB7	**Both**	**0.58**	**0.73**	**0.40**
33	Poor	255	Frank		0.67		
34	Poor	127	Survival BB8		0.60		
35	Poor	211	Rot Tawn 1180 ⁰	Lower	0.67	0.74	
36		57	BB8		0.61		
37		123	Joe	**Upper**	0.56		0.77

Shaded rows indicate the poor trackers.

Table 7.
List of optimal copulas for the 36 patients with each patient's WPB status, number of time points over ICU stay, copula type, values for copula tau (τ) for the main region, the lower or upper regions taus for the patient's (score, dose) bivariate profiles.

addition to the values for copula tau (τ) for the main region, the lower or upper regions, as applicable for the patients' (nurses' score, dose) bivariate profiles.

In regards to the distribution of copula types by WPB (good versus poor) tracking status, there are four Frank copula types of the 13 poor trackers, in comparison to 1 good tracker being a Frank copula type. Of the 23 good trackers, the majority are either Survival Gumbel (5 of these), Survival BB8 (5 such), or Gaussian (4) copula types (**Table 4**).

Furthermore, of the 23 good trackers, eight patients (35%) have bivariate dependence with a lower tail, 12 patients (52%) with no tails, 1 patient P32 (4.3%) with both upper and lower tails, and 2 (8.7%) (P23 and 27) with an upper tail. In comparison of the 13 poor trackers, there are four patients (31%) with a lower tail, seven (54%) with no tails, one patient P25 (7.7%) with both tails, and one patient 4 (7.7%) with an upper tail (**Table 4**).

Copulas that are unique to the poor trackers are the Survival BB7 (P32 with upper and lower tails, a poor tracker, displayed in **Figure** 7 and the Rotated Tawn type 1, 180^0 (P35 with an upper tail, a poor tracker displayed in **Figure 8**). Unique copula types found only for the good trackers are the Clayton (P3 and P19, each have lower tails), the BB8 (P30 and P36 both with no tails), the t copula (P25 with upper and lower tails) shown in **Figure 9** and the Joe copula (P37, upper tail) displayed in **Figure 10**.

3.2 Visuals, tail dependence, taus, dose/score thresholds of 10 patients

Details of equations, copulas and visualisations will focus on the following list of 10 patients given in **Tables 8 and 9**. Visualisations comprise patients' score and dose trajectories with associated 95% WPB bands, copula plots, K-plots, along with associated equations, relevant tau for tails and a clear delineation dose and nurses' score thresholds related to upper and lower tails, when they exist. Specifically lower and upper tail tau (τ) values, their percentile positions in the patient bivariate trajectories of length in ICU, associated lower and/or upper tail thresholds for the infusion dose and nurse's score threshold are given in **Table 8**. **Table 9** gives the associated equation parameters contrasting linear correlation (r) with our novel copula-tail based approach. **Figures 11** and **12** display the bivariate trajectories and 90% WPB bands of the patients. Full set of equations and tail thresholds are given in **Tables A.1** and **A.2** in the Appendix.

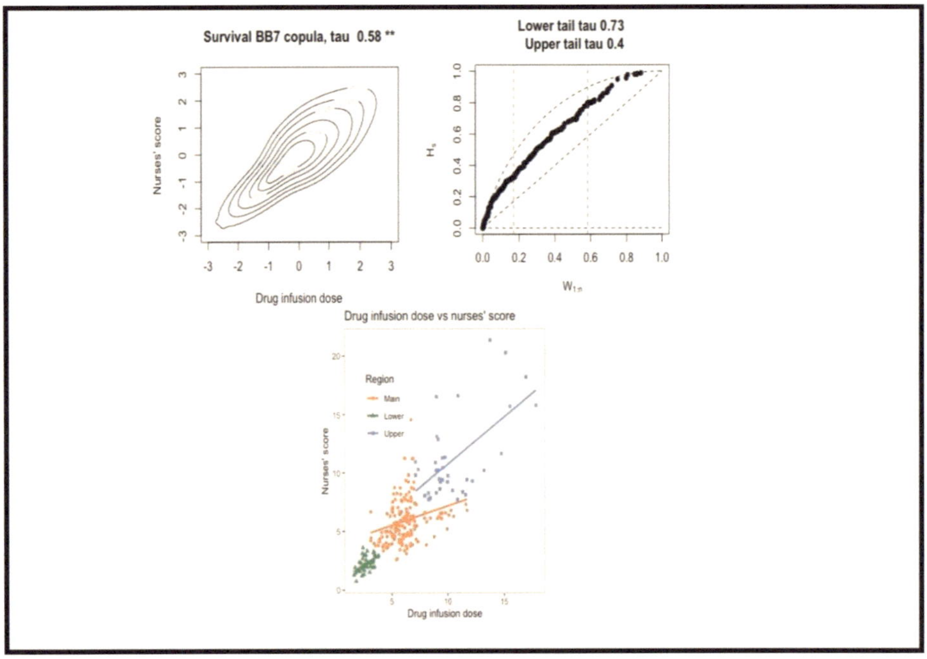

Figure 7.
P32 a poor tracker with 2 tails - copula plot, main tau, *K- plot and tail* taus *(upper panel); best fit line(s) (lower panel). LT* tau = 0.73, *UT* tau = 0.40, *(LT, UT) dose threshold = (3.90, 7.02), (LT, UT) score threshold = (3.62, 7.63).*

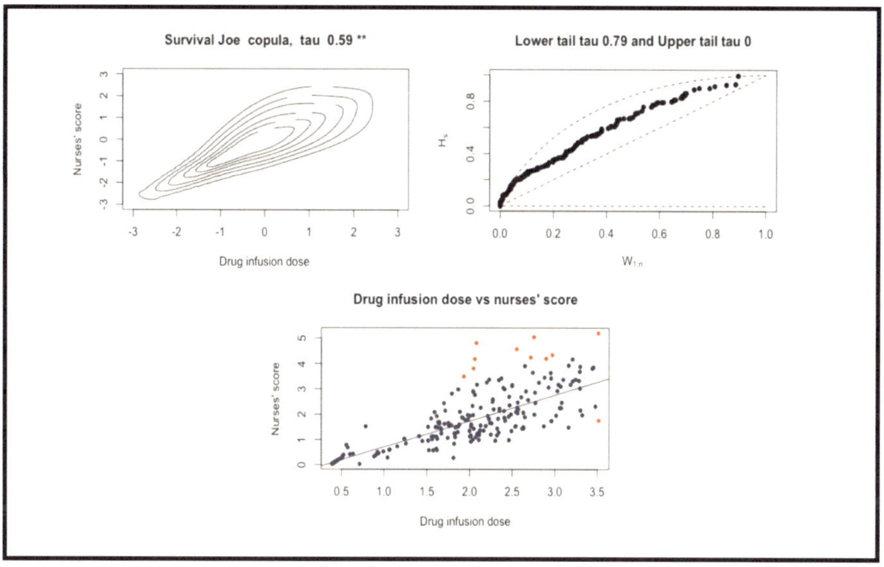

Figure 8.
P28 poor tracker with a lower tail - copula plot, main tau, *K- plot and tail* tau *(upper panel); best fit line(s) (lower panel) relating P28 nurses' score with dose. LT tail* tau *= 0.79, LT dose threshold = 1.70 and LT score threshold = 1.20.*

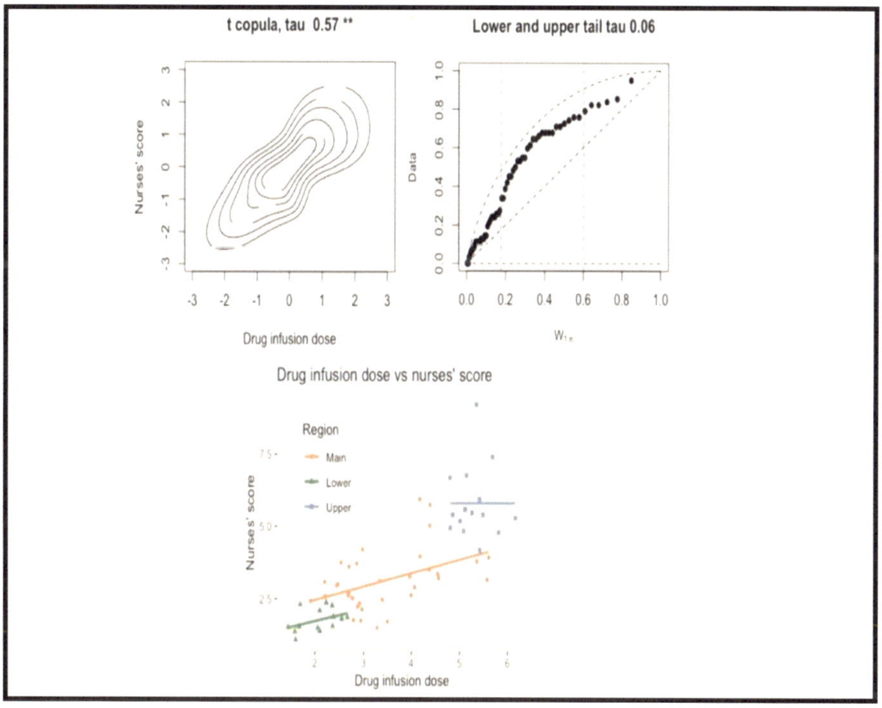

Figure 9.
P25 good tracker with 2 tails - copula plot, main region tau *K-plot, and tail* taus *(upper panel); best fit line(s) (lower panel) LT* tau *= 0.06, UT* tau *= 0.06, and (LT, UT) dose threshold = (2.68, 4.43), with (LT, UT) score threshold = (2.41, 3.94).*

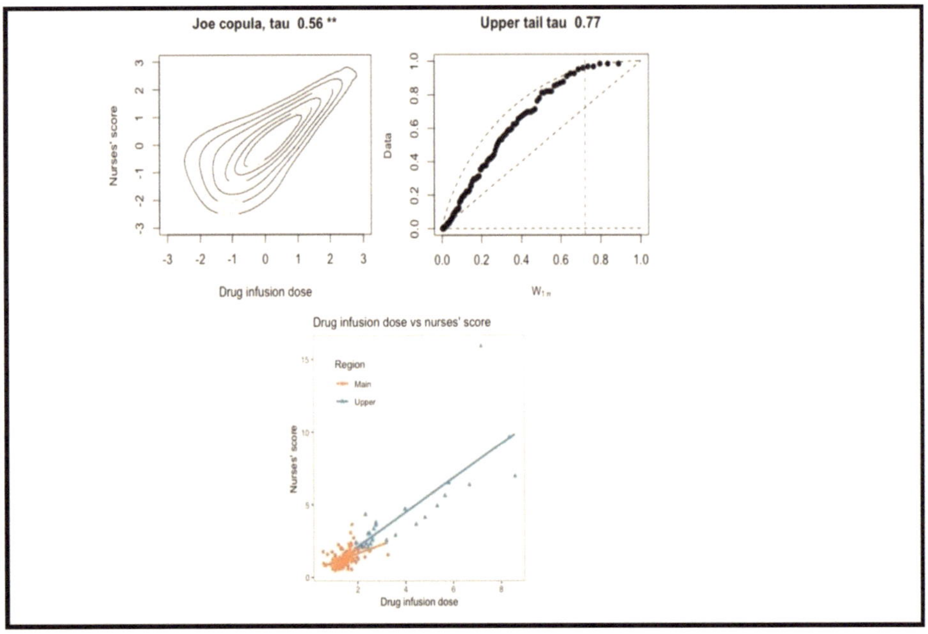

Figure 10.
P37 good tracker with upper tail - copula plot, main tau, *K- plot and tail* tau *(upper panel); best fit line(s) (lower panel) relating P37 nurses' A-S score with dose. UT* tau = *0.77, UT dose threshold* = *2.53, and UT nurse score threshold* = *2.99.*

			Lower Tail tau (τ)		Upper Tail tau (τ)		Dose threshold		Score threshold	
P no.	**Tails**	**n**	**n**	**Per centile**	**n**	**Per centile**	**Lower**	**Upper**	**Lower**	**Upper**
2	Lower	63	28	44.44			0.96		0.83	
4	Upper	63			15	76.19		2.82		2.75
15	Lower	63	22	34.92			3.47		3.05	
23	Upper	57			10	82.46		1.77		1.97
25	**Both tails**	**63**	**14**	**33.33**	**15**	**68.25**	**2.68**	**4.43**	**2.41**	**3.94**
27	**No tails**	223								
28	Lower	203	59	29.06			1.70		1.20	
32	**Both tails**	**252**	**44**	**20.64**	**38**	**74.60**	**3.90**	**7.02**	**3.62**	**7.63**
35	Lower	211	42	19.91			0.72		0.66	
37	Upper	123			17	86.18		2.53		2.99

Shaded rows are the poor trackers.

Table 8.
Upper and/or lower tail positions (percentiles) and associated lower/upper thresholds for dose and nurses' A-S score.

3.3 Prediction equation of score in relation to dose allowing tail dependence

In this subsection, we focus on 7 of the 10 selected patients reported in **Table 8**. Specifically, two patients with both lower and upper tails (P32 and P35), three

		Linear correlation (r)			Novel Regression (estimates)				adj R^2 quare	
P no.	**Tail status**	**Main region**	**Lower tail**	**Upper tail**	**Intercept**	**Dose Slope**	**Dose Slope Lower**	**Dose Slope Upper**	**Simple LR R^2**	**Novel method R^2**
2	Lower	0.39	0.77		0.27	0.85	−0.37		0.42	0.44
4	**Upper**	0.38		0.66	0.79	0.52		0.45	0.57	0.61
15	Lower	0.28	0.75		0.86	0.83	−0.34		0.45	0.47
23	**Upper**	0.51		0.62	0.34	0.58		0.52	0.64	0.68
25	**Both**	**0.44**	**0.41**	**0.00**	**1.55**	**0.46**	−0.35	**0.34**	**0.60**	**0.70**
27	None	0.84			−0.36	1.06			0.71	
28	Lower	0.46	0.84		0.008	0.97	−0.35		0.57	0.59
32	**Both**	**0.26**	**0.55**	**0.61**	**3.23**	**0.43**	−0.75	**0.33**	**0.60**	**0.67**
35	Lower	0.72	0.77		0.23	0.91	−0.79		0.63	0.64
37	**Upper**	0.54		0.75	0.17	0.78		0.32	0.74	0.75

Table 9.
Upper and/or lower tail dose relationships, equations, and associated change in adjusted R^2 for simple LR vs *our novel approach. Shaded rows indicate the poor trackers.*

patients with only upper tails (P4, P23, P37), and two patients with only lower tails (P2 and P15). For each of these seven patients, our novel equation relating each patient's nurses' agitation severity rank score versus the patient's infusion dose with parameter estimates and p-values is reported below. In addition, interpretation of the equations in regard to regions where the nurses' score either under or overestimates the patient's agitation with respect to so-called ground truth, this being the patient's automated infusion dose is reported per patient.

Patient 32 poor tracker, 2 tails, R^2 squared (non adj, adjusted) = (0.60, 0.67).

Score = 3.23 + 0.43Dose-0.75Dose*LT + 0.33Dose*UT (**Table 10**): The intercept of 3.23 indicates that the patient is experiencing severe "chronic" background agitation. The slope of 0.43 indicates that in the moderate agitation zone nurses tend to strongly underestimate the patient's agitation severity. In mild agitation zone, nurses tend to still underestimate the agitation severity. In severe agitation zone, nurses tend to overestimate the patient's agitation severity on average 0.33 points higher (**Figures 7** and **11**). For P32 LT *tau* = 0.73, UT *tau* = 0.40, and its bivariate (LT, UT) *dose* thresholds are (3.90, 7.02), with (LT, UT) *nurses' score* thresholds of (3.62, 7.63).

Patient 25 – good tracker, 2 tails, R^2 squared (non adj, adjusted) = (0.60, 0.70).

Score = 1.55 + 0.46Dose-0.35Dose*LT + 0.34Dose*UT (**Table 10**): The intercept of 1.55 indicates that the patient is experiencing "chronic" background agitation. The slope of 0.46 indicates that in the moderate agitation zone nurses tend to strongly underestimate the patient's agitation severity. In severe agitation zone, nurses tend to overestimate the agitation severity. In the mild agitation zone, nurses tend to assign a rating that is, on average, 0.35 points lower than expected for the patient's given agitation severity. In the severe agitation zone, nurses tend to overestimate the agitation severity on average, 0.34 points higher than expected for the patient's given agitation severity (**Figure 9**, see also **Figure 11**). For P25 LT tau = 0.06, UT tau = 0.06, and its (LT, UT) dose threshold = (2.68, 4.43), (LT, UT) *score* threshold of (2.41, 3.94).

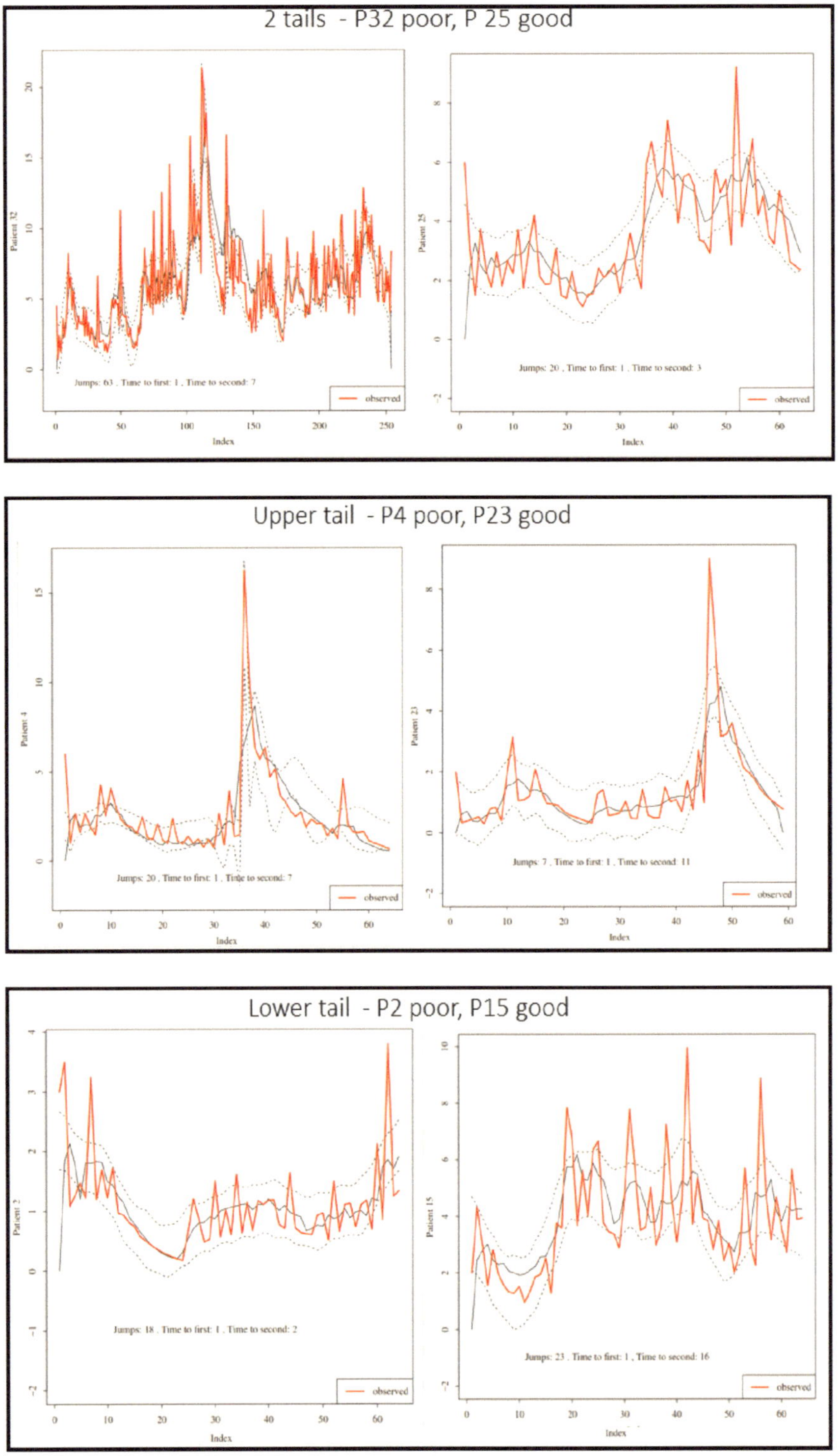

Figure 11.
Line plots of nurses' score (observed, red) and dose (black line), with 95% WPB bands for P32, P25 (both tails); P4, P23 (upper tail); P2, P15 (lower tail).

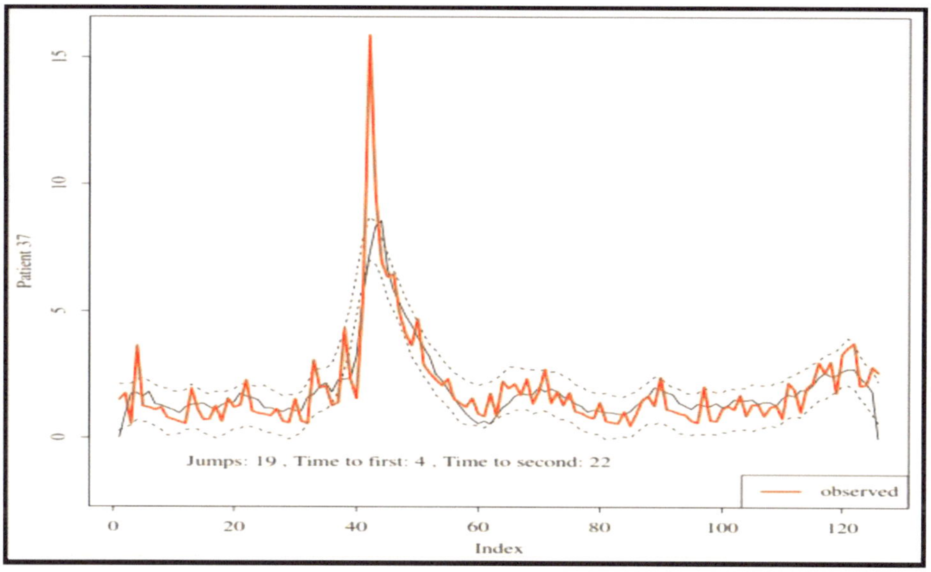

Figure 12.
Line plots of nurses' score (observed, red) vs. dose (black line), with 90% WPB bands for P37 good tracker.

Patient 32 - poor, 2 tails Adjusted R-squared: 0.66	**Estimate**	**Standard Error**	**t value**	**P value**	
Intercept	3.2342	0.5162	6.27	1.60E−09	***
Dose	0.4285	0.0828	5.18	4.70E−07	***
Dose*LT	−0.7506	0.1503	−4.99	1.10E−06	***
Dose*UT	0.3309	0.0497	6.65	1.80E−10	***
Patient 25 - good, 2 tails Adjusted R-squared: 0.70	Estimate	Standard Error	t value	P value	
Intercept	1.5481	0.5503	2.81	0.0067	**
Dose	0.4603	0.1543	2.98	0.0042	**
Dose*LT	−0.3475	0.1719	−2.02	0.0477	*
Dose*UT	0.3424	0.0788	4.34	5.60E-05	***

		Linear correlation (r)			**Novel Regression (estimates)**				**adj R^2 quare**	
P no.	Tail status	Main region	Lower tail	Upper tail	**Intercept**	**Dose Slope**	**Dose Slope Lower**	**Dose Slope Upper**	Simple LR R^2	**Novel method R^2**
32	**Both**	0.26	0.55	0.61	3.23	0.43	−0.75	0.33	0.60	0.67
25	**Both**	0.44	0.41	0.00	1.55	0.46	−0.35	0.34	0.60	0.70

Patient 4 poor tracker, UT R^2 squared (non adj, adjusted) = (0.57, 0.61).

Table 10.
P32 equation, poor tracker with 2 tails and LT tau = *0.73, UT* tau = *0.40. P25 equation, poor tracker with 2 tails and LT* tau = *0.06, UT* tau = *0.06.*

Score = 0.79 + 0.52Dose+0.45Dose*UT (**Table 11**): The slope of 0.52 indicates that in the moderate agitation zone nurses tend to strongly underestimate the patient'sagitation severity. In the severe agitation zone, nurses tend to overestimate the agitation severity. There are 14 (out of a total of 63) such occurrences indicating that approximately only one in every four ratings, nurses tend to overestimate patients' agitation severity (**Figure 13**, see also **Figure 11**). For P4 UT *tau* = 0.69, and its UT dose threshold = 2.82 and UT nurses' score threshold = 2.75.

Patient 23 good tracker, UT R^2 squared (non adj, adjusted) = (0.64, 0.68).

Score = 0.34 + 0.58Dose+0.52Dose*UT (**Table 11**): The slope of 0.58 indicates that in the moderate agitation zone nurses tend to strongly underestimate the patient's agitation severity. In periods of severe agitation, nurses tend to overestimate the agitation severity. There are 10 (out of a total of 57) such occurrences indicating that approximately only one in every five ratings, nurses tend to overestimate patient 23's agitation (**Figure 14**, see also **Figure 11**). For P23 UT *tau* = 0.68, and its UT dose threshold = 1.77 and UT nurses' score threshold = 1.97.

Patient 37 good tracker, UT R^2 squared (non adj, adjusted) = (0.74, 0.75).

Patient 4 - poor, Upper Tail Score = 0.17+ 0.78Dose+0.32Dose*UT (**Table 11**): The slope of 0.78 indicates that in the moderate agitation zone nurses tend to moderately

Patient 4 - poor, Upper Tail **Adjusted R-squared: 0.61**	**Estimate**	**Standard Error**	**t value**	**P value**	
Intercept	0.79	0.446	1.77	0.082	.
Dose	0.521	0.238	2.19	0.032	*
Dose*UT	0.445	0.189	2.35	0.022	*
Patient 23 - good, Upper Tail Adjusted R-squared: 0.68	Estimate	Standard Error	t value	P value	
Intercept	0.343	0.257	1.34	0.187	NS
Dose	0.576	0.24	2.4	0.0199	*
Dose*UT	0.524	0.196	2.68	0.0098	**
Patient 37 - good, Upper Tail Adjusted R-squared: 0.75	Estimate	Standard Error	t value	P value	
Intercept	0.165	0.273	0.61	0.546	NS
Dose	0.778	0.186	4.18	5.60E−05	***
Dose*UT	0.318	0.143	2.23	0.028	*

		Linear correlation (r)			**Novel Regression (estimates)**				**adj R^2 quare**	
P no.	Tail status	Main region	Lower tail	Upper tail	**Intercept**	**Dose Slope**	**Dose Slope Lower**	**Dose Slope Upper**	Simple LR R^2	**Novel method R^2**
4	Upper	0.38		0.66	0.79	0.52		0.45	0.57	0.61
23	Upper	0.51		0.62	0.34	0.58		0.52	0.64	0.68
37	Upper	0.54		0.75	0.17	0.78		0.32	0.74	0.75

Table 11.
P4 equation, poor tracker with upper tail and UT tau = *0.69. P23 equation, poor tracker with upper tail and UT* tau = *0.68.*

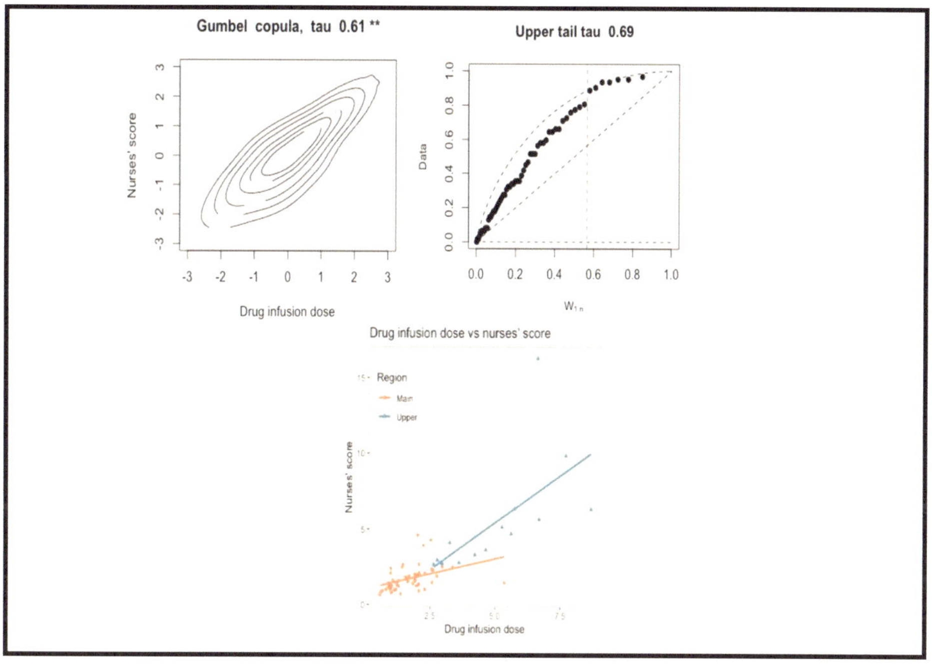

Figure 13.
P4 poor tracker with upper tail - copula plot, main tau, *K- plot and tail* tau *(upper panel); best fit line(s) (lower panel) relating P4 nurses' A-S score with dose. UT* tau = *0.69, UT dose threshold* = *2.82 and UT nurse score threshold* = *2.75.*

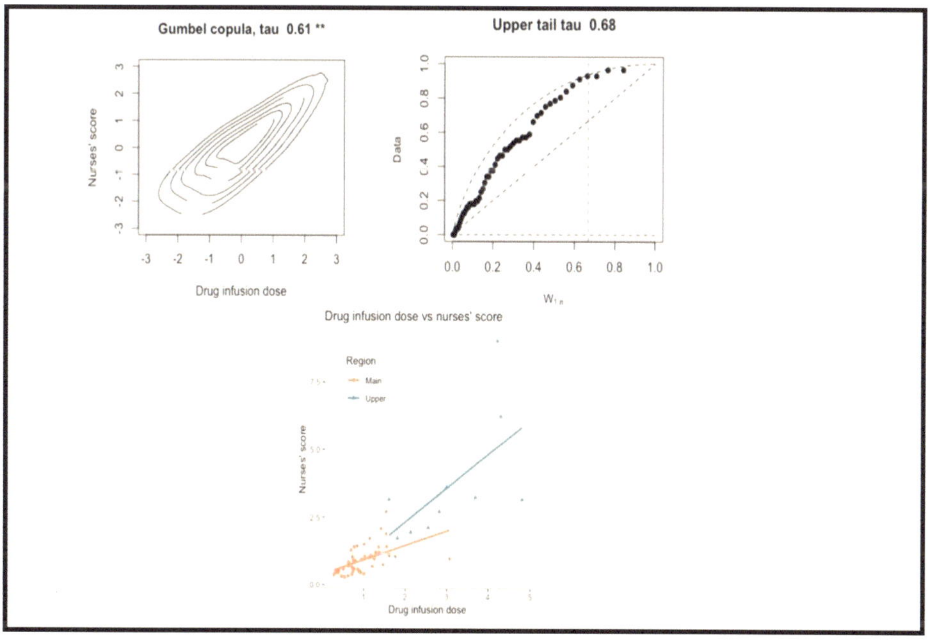

Figure 14.
P23 good tracker with upper tail - copula plot, main tau, *K- plot and tail* tau *(upper panel); best fit line(s) (lower panel) relating P23 nurses' A-S score with dose. UT* tau = *0.68, UT dose threshold* = *1.77 and UT nurse score threshold* = *1.97.*

underestimate the patient's agitation severity. In the patient's severe agitation zone, nurses tend to overestimate agitation severity. There are 25 (out of a total of 123) such occurrences indicating that approximately only in one in every five ratings, nurses tend to overestimate patients' agitation severity accurately. (**Figure 10**, see also **Figure 12**). For P37 UT tau = 0.77, and its UT dose threshold = 2.53 and UT nurses' score threshold = 2.99.

P37 equation, good tracker with upper tail and UT *tau* = 0.77.

Patient 2 poor tracker, LT R^2 squared (non adj, adjusted) = (0.42, 0.44).

Score = 0.27 + 0.85Dose - 0.37Dose*LT (**Table 12**): The slope of 0.85 indicates that in the moderate agitation zone nurses tend to underestimate the patient's agitation severity. In the mild agitation zone, nurses tend to assign a rating that is, on average, 0.37 points lower than expected for the patient's given agitation severity. There are 28 out of a total of 63 such occurrences indicating that in around one in every two ratings, nurses tend to underestimate agitation severity (**Figure 15**, also **Figure 11**).

Patient 15 good tracker, LT R^2 squared (non adj, adjusted) = (0.45, 0.47).

Score = 0.86 + 0.83Dose - 0.34Dose*LT (**Table 12**): The slope of 0.83 indicates that in the moderate agitation zone nurses tend to underestimate the patient's agitation severity accurately. In the mild agitation zone, nurses tend to underestimate the patient's agitation severity even more. There are 22 (out of a total of 43) such occurrences indicating that approximately one in every three ratings, nurses tend to *strongly* underestimate the patients' agitation severity (**Figure 16**, see also **Figure 11**).

Patient 28 poor tracker, LT R^2 squared (non adj, adjusted) = (0.57, 0.59)
Score = 0.01 + 0.97Dose-0.35Dose*LT (**Table 13**).

The slope of 0.97 indicates that in the moderate agitation zone nurses tend to estimate the patient's agitation severity fairly accurately. In the mild agitation zone, however,

Patient 2 - poor, Lower Tail **Adjusted R-squared: 0.44**	**Estimate**	**Standard Error**	**t value**	**P value**	
Intercept	0.269	0.208	1.29	0.201	NS
Dose	0.85	0.158	5.36	1.40E−06	***
Dose*LT	−0.367	0.184	−1.99	0.052	.
Patient 15 - good, Lower Tail Adjusted R-squared: 0.47	Estimate	Standard Error	t value	P value	
Intercept	0.861	0.962	0.9	0.37412	NS
Dose	0.834	0.206	4.05	0.00015	***
Dose*LT	−0.344	0.177	−1.94	0.05664	.

		Linear correlation (r)			**Novel Regression (estimates)**				**adj R^2 quare**	
P no.	Tail status	Main region	Lower tail	Upper tail	**Intercept**	**Dose Slope**	**Dose Slope Lower**	**Dose Slope Upper**	Simple LR $\mathbf{R^2}$	**Novel method $\mathbf{R^2}$**
2	Lower	0.39	0.77		0.27	0.85	−0.37		0.42	0.44
15	Lower	0.28	0.75		0.86	0.83	−0.34		0.45	0.47

Table 12.
P2 equation, poor tracker with lower tail and LT tau = *0.64. P15 equation, good tracker with lower tail and LT* tau = *0.74.*

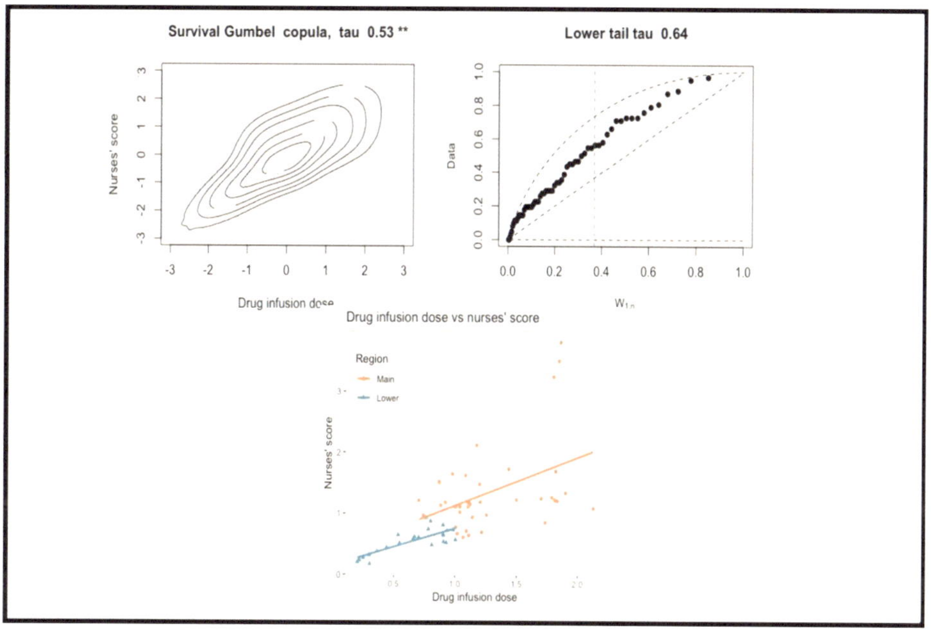

Figure 15.
P2 poor tracker with lower tail - copula plot, main tau, *K- plot and tail* tau *(upper panel); best fit line(s) (lower panel) relating P2 nurses' A-S score with dose. LT* tau *= 0.64, with LT dose threshold = 0.96 and LT nurses' score threshold = 0.83.*

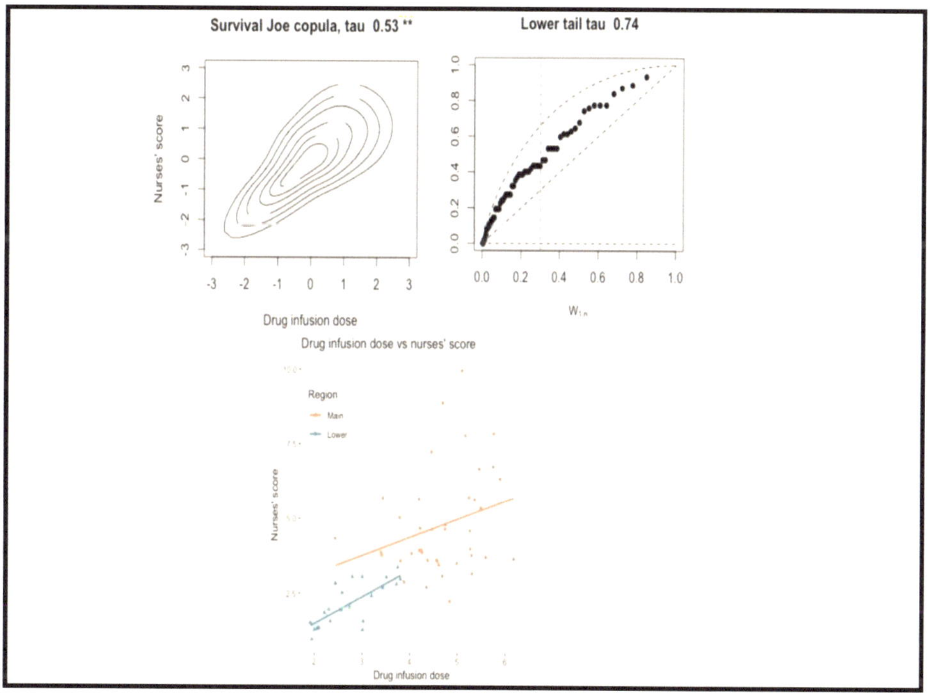

Figure 16.
P15 good tracker with lower tail - copula plot, main tau, *K- plot and tail* tau *(upper panel); best fit line(s) (lower panel) relating P15 nurses' A-S score with dose. LT tail* tau *= 0.74, LT dose threshold = 3.47 and LT score threshold = 3.05.*

Patient 28 – poor, Lower Tail	**Estimate**	**Standard Error**	***t*-value**	***P*-value**	**adj R^2 = 0.64**
Intercept	0.00876	0.17549	0.05	0.96023	
Dose	0.96582	0.07356	13.13	< 2e−16	***
Dose*LT	−0.345	0.1014	−3.4	0.00081	***
Patient 35 – poor, Lower Tail	Estimate Std.	Error t	t value	P value	adj R^2 = 0.644
Intercept	0.2322	0.1128	2.06	0.04084	*
Dose	0.9097	0.0597	15.24	< 2e−16	***
Dose*LT	−0.7898	0.2253	−3.51	0.00056	***
Patient 27 – poor, no tails	Estimate Std.	Error t	t value	P value	adj R^2 = 0.71
Intercept	−0.3644	0.2062	−1.77	0.079	.
Dose	1.061	0.0453	23.4	<2e-16	***

		Linear correlation (r)			Novel Regression (estimates)				adj R^2 quare	
P no.	Tail status	Main region	Lower tail	Upper tail	Intercept	Dose Slope	Dose Slope Lower	Dose Slope Upper	Simple LR R^2	Novel method R^2
28	Lower	0.46	0.84		0.00	0.97	−0.35		0.57	0.59
35	Lower	0.72	0.77		0.23	0.91	−0.79		0.63	0.64
27	None	0.84			−0.36	1.06			0.71	

Table 13.
P28 equation, poor tracker with lower tail LT tau = *0.79. P35 equation, poor tracker with lower tail LT* tau = *0.74. P27 equation, poor tracker no tails.,* tau = *0.78 (**Figures 18** and **19**).*

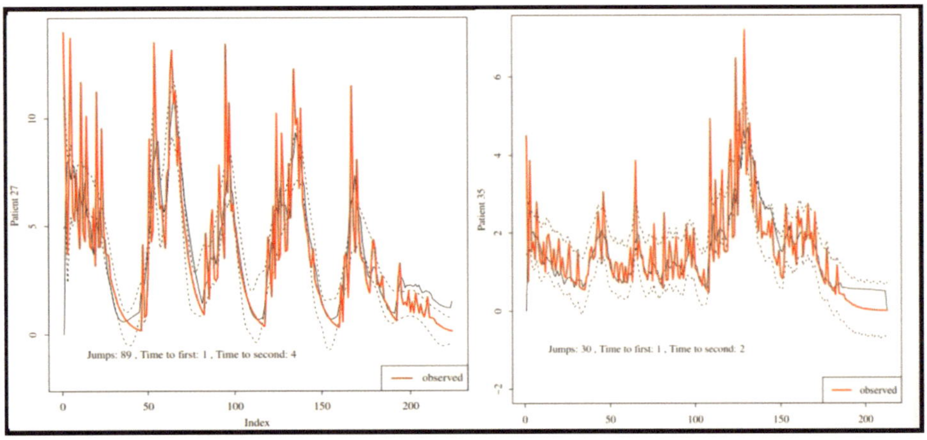

Figure 17.
Line plots of nurses' score (observed, red) vs. dose (black line), with 95% WPB bands for P27 and P35 poor trackers with and P27 poor tracker with no tails.

nurses tend to underestimate patient 28's agitation severity more. There are 29 (out of a total of 203) such occurrences indicating that one in every seven ratings, nurses tend to strongly underestimate patients' agitation severity (**Figure 17**, see also **Figure 18**).

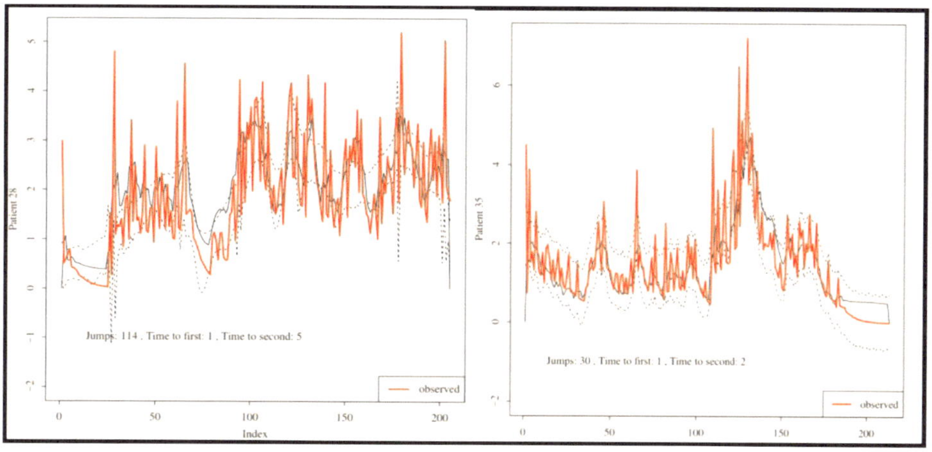

Figure 18.
Line plots of nurses' score (observed, red) vs. dose (black line), with 95% WPB bands for P28 and P35 both poor trackers with lower tails.

Patient 35 poor tracker, LT R^2 squared (non adj, adjusted) = (0.63, 0.64)
Score = 0.23 + 0.91Dose-0.79Dose*LT (**Table 13**): The intercept of 0.23 indicates that the patient is experiencing mild "chronic" background agitation. The slope of 0.91 indicates that in the moderate agitation zone nurses tend to slightly underestimate the patient's agitation severity. In the mild agitation zone, nurses tend to *strongly* underestimate the patient's agitation severity even more. There are 42 (out of a total of 211) such occurrences indicating that approximately one in every five ratings, nurses tend to underestimate patients' agitation severity (**Figures 8** and **18**).

4. Conclusions

Copulas were successfully implemented to capture non-linear dependence, and establish the presence of lower (LT) and/or upper tail (UT) dependence between the nurses' A-S rating and the automated sedation dose (**Figure 20**). Establishing the presence of tail dependence and patient-specific lower and/or upper thresholds for areas with different agitation intensities has significant implications for effective administration of sedatives. Copulas unique to the poor trackers were the Survival BB7 and Rotated Tawn type 1, 180. Unique copula types of the good trackers were Clayton, BB8, and t copula. To the best fit copulas, we established for each patients' bivariate score and dose trajectories regions of mild, moderate, and severe agitation and their lower and upper tail thresholds, if any, in the dependence, relationship via K-plots and our novel equation relating patient's nurses' score to dose. We found that for lower tail dependence, nurses tend to underestimate the patient's agitation in the moderate agitation zone. In the mild agitation zone, nurses tend to assign a rating that is, on average, 0.30 to 0.45 points lower than expected for the patient's given agitation. For upper tail dependence nurses tend to either moderately or strongly underestimate patient's agitation in the moderate agitation zone; but in periods of severe agitation, tend to overestimate a patient's agitation. When both lower and upper tails exist, nurses tend to strongly underestimate agitation in the moderate zone and then tend to still underestimate agitation in mild agitation periods; but in the severe zone nurses tend to overestimate agitation on average by 0.34 points. We also determined the

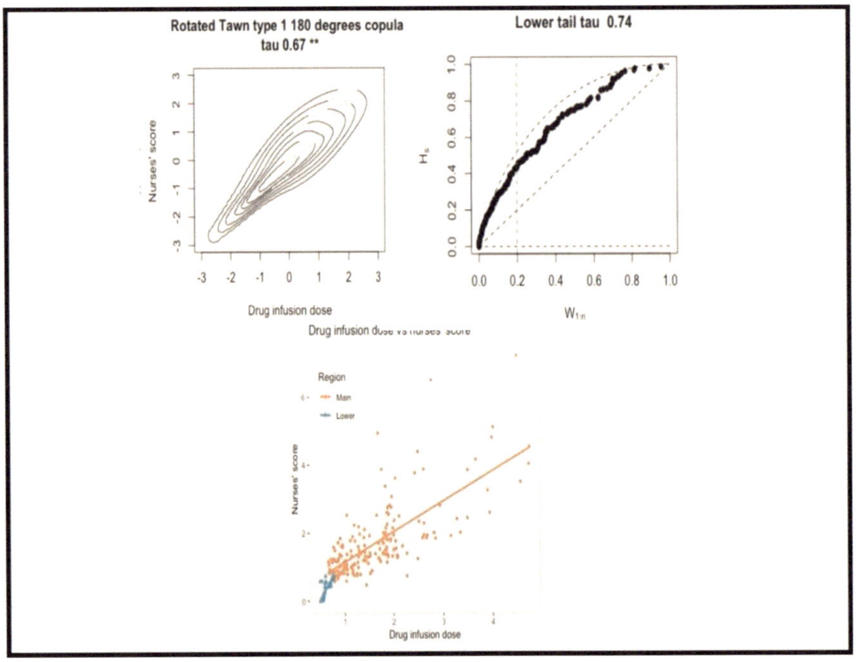

Figure 19.
P35 poor tracker with a lower tail - copula plot, main tau, *K- plot and tail* tau *(upper panel); best fit line(s) (lower panel) relating P35 nurses' score with dose. LT tail* tau = *0.74, LT dose threshold = 0.72 and LT score threshold = 0.66.*

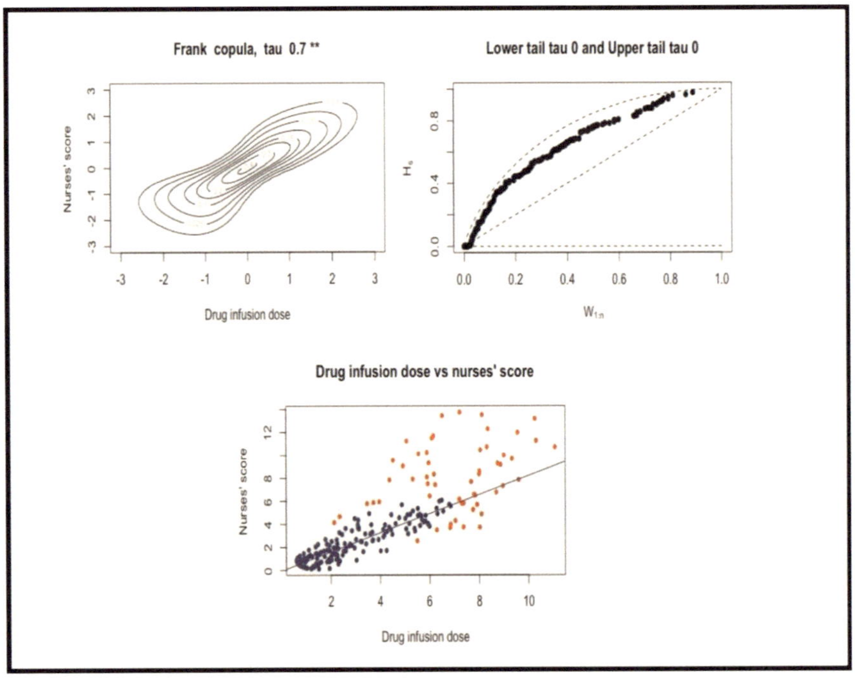

Figure 20.
P27 poor tracker with no tails- copula plot, main tau = *0.70, K- plot and tail* tau *(upper panel); best fit line (lower panel) relating P27 nurses' score with dose.*

DOI: http://dx.doi.org/10.5772/intechopen.105753

number of occurrences over the patient's total ICU stay, where nurses tend to under/over- estimate agitation. Finding thresholds and regions of mismatch between the nurses' scores and sedation dose potentially provides a way to improved alerting systems for over/under-sedation. Our approach lends credence to augmenting conventional RASS and SAS agitation measures with semi-automated systems and identifying thresholds and regions of deviance for alerting increased risk.

A. Appendix

			Lower Tail tau (τ)		Upper Tail tau (τ)		Dose threshold		Nurses' Score threshold	
P no.	**Tails**	**n**	**n**	**Per centile**	**n**	**Per centile**	**Lower**	**Upper**	**Lower**	**Upper**
1	Lower	59	19	32.20			0.52		0.38	
2	Lower	63	28	44.44			0.96		0.83	
3	Lower	63		22.22			1.35		1.31	
4	Upper	63			15	76.19		2.82		2.75
5	Lower	48	17	35.40			1.25		1.06	
6	Lower	63	23	36.51			1.38		1.23	
7	Lower	63	8	12.70			0.44		0.15	
8	Lower	127	33	25.98			3.02		2.57	
10		255								
11		111								
12		127								
13		63								
14	Lower	49	20	40.82			0.96		0.82	
15	Lower	63	22	34.92			3.47		3.05	
16		127								
17		63								
18		63								
19	Lower	127	28	22.04			6.46		5.23	
20		127								
21		61								
22		127								
23	**Upper**	57			10	82.46		1.77		1.97
24		127								
25	**Both**	**63**	**14**	**33.33**	**15**	**68.25**	2.68	4.43	2.41	3.94
26		63								
27		223								
28	Lower	203	59	29.06			1.70		1.20	
29		53								

			Lower Tail tau (τ)		Upper Tail tau (τ)	Dose threshold			Nurses' Score threshold	
P no.	**Tails**	**n**	**n**	**Per centile**	**n**	**Per centile**	**Lower**	**Upper**	**Lower**	**Upper**
30		60								
31		255								
32	**Both**	**252**	**44**	**20.64**	**38**	**74.60**	3.90	7.02	3.62	7.63
33		255								
34		127								
35	Lower	211	42	19.91			0.72		0.66	
36		57								
37	**Upper**	123			17	86.18		2.53		2.99

Shaded rows are the poor trackers.

Table A.1.
List of copulas and upper and/or lower tail positions (percentiles) and associated lower/upper thresholds for dose and nurses' A-S score.

		Linear correlation (r)			Novel Regression (estimates)				adj R^2	
P no.	**Tail status**	**Main region**	**Lower tail**	**Upper tail**	**Intercept**	**Dose Slope**	**Dose Slope Lower**	**Dose Slope Upper**	**Simple LR R^2**	**Novel method R^2**
1	Lower	0.44	0.81		0.152	0.84	−0.46		0.49	0.53
2	Lower	0.39	0.77		0.27	0.85	−0.37		0.42	0.44
3	Lower	0.36	0.65		0.91	0.58	−0.50		0.30	0.34
4	**Upper**	0.38		0.66	0.79	0.52		0.45	0.57	0.61
5	Lower	0.21	0.75		0.49	0.75	−0.45		0.33	0.39
6	Lower	0.37	0.56		0.66	0.68	−0.36		0.36	0.41
7	Lower	0.85	0.99		−0.22	1.17	−0.45		0.77	0.77
8	Lower	0.64	0.76		0.01	1.01	−0.29		0.62	0.63
10		0.82			−0.51	1.19			0.67	
11		0.83			−0.19	1.21			0.68	
12		0.68			0.18	0.94			0.46	
13		0.87			−0.43	1.12			0.75	
14	Lower	0.50	0.70		0.11	0.95	−0.40		0.61	0.64
15	Lower	0.28	0.75		0.86	0.83	−0.34		0.45	0.47
16		0.81			−0.17	1.03			0.66	
17		0.71			0.19	0.90			0.50	
18		0.77			0.01	1.06			0.58	
19	Lower	0.47	0.55		0.80	0.94	−0.34		0.48	0.50
20		0.70			−0.31	1.16			0.49	
21		0.74			−0.10	1.08			0.55	

		Linear correlation (r)			Novel Regression (estimates)				adj R^2	
P no.	**Tail status**	**Main region**	**Lower tail**	**Upper tail**	**Intercept**	**Dose Slope**	**Dose Slope Lower**	**Dose Slope Upper**	**Simple LR R^2**	**Novel method R^2**
22		0.77			−0.58	1.16			0.59	
23	**Upper**	0.51		0.62	0.34	0.58		0.52	0.64	0.68
24		0.78			−0.50	1.14			0.60	
25	**Both**	**0.44**	**0.41**	**0.00**	**1.55**	**0.46**	−0.35	**0.34**	**0.60**	**0.70**
26		0.78			−0.07	1.08			0.61	
27		0.84			−0.36	1.06			0.71	
28	Lower	0.46	0.84		0.008	0.97	−0.35		0.57	0.59
29		0.86			0.24	0.89			0.73	
30		0.55			−0.04	1.04			0.29	
31		0.79			1.00	1.16			0.63	
32	**Both**	**0.26**	**0.55**	**0.61**	**3.23**	**0.43**	−0.75	**0.33**	**0.60**	**0.67**
33		0.83			−0.98	1.23			0.68	
34		0.74			-9.23	1.06			0.55	
35	Lower	0.72	0.77		0.23	0.91	−0.79		0.63	0.64
36		0.86			−0.45	1.11		0.28	0.73	
37	**Upper**	0.54		0.75	0.17	0.78		0.32	0.74	0.75

Shaded rows indicate the poor trackers. Boxes regarding indicate largest differences between R^2 equation fit.

Table A.2.
Upper and/or lower tail dose relationships, equations, and associated change in adjusted R^2 for simple LR vs *our novel approach.*

Author details

Irene Hudson[1]*, Ainura Tursunalieva[2] and J. Geoffrey Chase[3]

1 Mathematical Sciences, School of Science, RMIT, Melbourne, Australia

2 Banking and Finance, Monash University, Melbourne, Australia

3 University of Canterbury, Christchurch, New Zealand

*Address all correspondence to: irene.hudson@rmit.edu.au

References

[1] Varndell W, Fry M, Elliot D. Emergency nurses' perceptions of sedation management practices for critically ill intubated patients: A qualitative study. Journal of Clinical Nursing. 2015;**24**(21–22): 3286-3895. DOI: 10.1111/jocn.12932

[2] Varndell W, Fry M, Elliot D. The validity, reliability, responsiveness and applicability of observation sedation-scoring instruments for use with adult patients in the emergency department: A systematic literature review. Australasian Emergency Nursing Journal. 2015;**18**(1):1-23. DOI: 10.1016/j.aenj.2014.07.001

[3] Sessler CN, Gosnell MS, Grap MJ, Brophy GM, O'Neal PV, Keane KA, et al. The Richmond agitation-sedation scale: Validity and reliability in adult intensive care unit patients. American Journal of Respiratory and Critical Care Medicine. 2002;**166**(1):1338-1344. DOI: 10.1164/rccm.2107138

[4] Fraser GL, Riker RR. Monitoring sedation, agitation, analgesia, and delirium in critically ill adult patients. Critical Care Clinics. 2001;**17**(4): 967-987. DOI: 10.1016/s0749-0704(05)70189-5

[5] Hochberg U, Sharon H, Bahir I, Brill S. Pain management - a Decade's perspective of a new subspecialty. Journal of pain. Research. 2021; **14**:923-930. DOI: 10.2147/JPR.S303815

[6] Pretorius A, Searle J, Marshall B. Barriers and enablers to emergency department nurses' management of patients' pain. Pain Management Nursing. 2015;**16**(3):372-379. DOI: 10.1016/j.pmn.2014.08.015

[7] Rashidi M, Molavynejad S, Javadi N, Adineh M, Sharhani A, Poursangbur T. The effect of using Richmond agitation and sedation (RASS) scale on hospital stay, ventilator dependence, and mortality rate in ICU inpatients: A randomised clinical trial. Journal of Research in Nursing. 2020;**25**(8): 734-746. DOI: 10.1177/1744987120943921

[8] Bush SH, Grassau PA, Yarmo MN, Zhang T, Zinkie SJ, Pereira JL. The Richmond agitation-sedation scale modified for palliative care inpatients (RASS-PAL): A pilot study exploring validity and feasibility in clinical practice. BMC Palliative Care. 2014; **13**(17):1-9

[9] Rudge AD, Chase JG, Shaw GM, Lee D. Physiological modelling of agitation-sedation dynamics including endogenous agitation reduction. Medical Engineering and Physics. 2006;**28**(7): 629-638. DOI: 10.1016/j.medengphy.2005.10.008

[10] Kang I, Hudson IL, Rudge A, Chase JG. Wavelet signatures and diagnostics for the assessment of ICU agitation-sedation protocols. In: Olkkonen H, editor. Discrete Wavelet Transforms. 1st ed. Rijeka: IntechOpen; 2011. pp. 321-348. DOI: 10.5772/20547

[11] Kang I, Hudson IL, Rudge A, Chase JG. Density estimation and wavelet Thresholding via Bayesian methods: A wavelet probability band and related metrics approach to assess agitation and sedation in ICU patients. In: Al-Asmari A, editor. Discrete Wavelet Transforms: A Compendium of New Approaches and Recent Applications. 1st ed. Rijeka: IntechOpen; 2013. pp. 127-162. DOI: 10.5772/52434

[12] Rudge AD, Chase JG, Shaw GM, Lee D, Wake GC, Hudson IL, et al. Impact of control on agitation-sedation dynamics. Control Engineering Practice. 2005;**13**(9):1139-1149. DOI: 10.1016/j.conengprac.2004.10.010

[13] Rudge AD, Chase JG, Shaw GM, Lee D, Hann CE. Parameter identification and sedative sensitivity analysis of an agitation-sedation model. Computer Methods and Programs in Biomedicine. 2006;**83**(3):211-221. DOI: 10.1016/j.cmpb.2006.06.011

[14] Chase JG, Rudge AD, Shaw GM, Wake GC, Lee D, Hudson IL. Modeling and control of the agitation-sedation cycle for critical care patients. Medical Engineering and Physics. 2004;**26**(6): 459-471. DOI: 10.1016/j.medengphy.2004.02.001

[15] Nikoloulopoulos AK, Joe H, Li H. Vine copulas with asymmetric tail dependence and applications to financial return data. Computational Statistics & Data Analysis. 2013;**56**(11):3659-3673. DOI: 10.1016/j.csda.2010.07.016

[16] Patton AJ. A review of copula models for economic time series. Journal of Multivariate Analysis. 2012;**110**:4-18. DOI: 10.1016/j.jmva.2012.02.021

[17] Winkelmann R. Copula bivariate probit models: With an application to medical expenditures. Health Economics. 2012;**21**(12):1444-1455. DOI: 10.1002/hec.1801

[18] Frees EW, Valdez EA. Understanding relationships using copulas. North American Actuarial Journal. 1998;**2**(1):1-25. DOI: 10.1080/10920277.1998.10595667

[19] Otani Y, Imai J. Pricing portfolio credit derivatives with stochastic recovery and systematic factor. IAENG International Journal of Applied Mathematics. 2013;**43**(4):176-184. http://www.iaeng.org/IJAM/issues_v43/issue_4/IJAM_43_4_02.pdf

[20] Tursunalieva A, Hudson I, Chase J. 'Copula modelling of nurses' agitation-sedation rating of ICU patients: Towards monitoring and health alerting tools'. In: Proceedings from the 23rd International Congress on Modelling and Simulation. Sondoss Elsawah (ed.). Melbourne, Australia: Modelling & Simulation Society of Australia & New Zealand (MSSANZ); 2019. pp. 835-841. https://mssanz.org.au/modsim2019/I4/tursunalieva.pdf 23]

[21] Tursunalieva A, Hudson I, Chase J. Copula modelling of nurses' agitation-sedation rating of ICU patients. In: Communications in Computer and Information Science. Simone Diniz Junqueira Barbosa, et al (ed.). vol. 1150. H. Nguyen (Ed.). Singapore: Springer Nature Singapore Pte Ltd.: 2019. pp. 148–161. DOI: 10.1007/978-981-15-1960-4_11

[22] Hudson IL. Modelling agitation-sedation (A-S) in ICU: An empirical transition and time to event analysis of poor and good tracking between nurses scores and automated A-S measures. In: Vargas-De-León C, editor. Biostatistics. Ist ed. Rijeka: InTechOpen; 2022 (in press)

[23] Bai J, Perron P. Computation and analysis of multiple structural change models. Journal of Applied Econometrics. 2003;**18**(1):1-22. DOI: 10.1002/jae.659

[24] Olson Dai Wai M, Zomorodi MG, James ML, Cox CE, Moretti EW, Riemen KE, et al. Exploring the impact of augmenting sedation assessment with physiologic monitors. Australian Critical Care. 2014;**27**(3):145-150. DOI: 10.1016/J.AUCC.2013.09.001

[25] Barbato M, Barclay G, Potter J, Yeo W, Chung J. Correlation between observational scales of sedation and comfort and bispectral index scores. Journal of Pain and Symptom Management. 2017;**54**:186-193

[26] West N, McBeth PB, Brodie SM, van Heusden K, Sunderland S, Ga D, et al. Feasibility of continuous sedation monitoring in critically ill intensive care unit patients using the Neuro SENSE WAV $_{CNS}$ index. Journal of Clinical Monitoring and Computing. 2018;**32**(6): 1081-1091. DOI: 10.1007/s10877-018-0115-6

[27] Genest C, Favre AC. Everything you always wanted to know about copula modeling but were afraid to ask. Journal of Hydrologic Engineering. 2007;**12**(4): 347-368. DOI: 10.1061/(ASCE) 1084-0699(2007)12:4(347)

[28] Joe H. Dependence Modeling with Copulas. 1st ed. Boca Raton: CRC Press; 2015 480 p. https://www.routledge.com/Dependence-Modeling-with-Copulas/Joe/p/book/9781466583221

[29] Boateng MA, Omari-Sasu AY, Avuglah RK, Frempong NK. A mixture of Clayton, Gumbel, and Frank copulas: A complete dependence model. Journal of Probability and Statistics. 2022;**2022**: 1-7. DOI: 10.1155/2022/1422394

[30] Clayton DG. A model for association in bivariate life tables and its application in epidemiological studies of familial tendency in chronic disease incidence. Biometrika. 1978;**65**(1):141-151. DOI: 10.2307/2335289

[31] Frank MJ. On the simultaneous associativity of F (x,y) and x+y-F (x,y). Aequationes mathematicae. 1979;**19**: 194-226. DOI: 10.1007/BF01844082

[32] Gumbel EJ. Bivariate exponential distributions. Journal of the American Statistical Association. 1960;**55**(292): 698-707. DOI: 10.2307/2281591

[33] Genest C, Boies JC. Detecting dependence with Kendall plots. Amer. Statist. 2004;**57**(4):275-284. DOI: 10.1198/0003130032431

[34] Vexler A, Afendras G, Markatou M. Multi-panel Kendall plot in light of an ROC curve analysis applied to measuring dependence. Statistics. 2019;**53**(2): 417-439. DOI: 10.1080/02331888.2018.1555586

[35] Kendall MG. A new measure of rank correlation. Biometrika. 1938;**30**(1–2): 81-93. DOI: 10.2307/2332226

Chapter 5

Bayesian Multilevel Modeling in Dental Research

Edilberta Tino-Salgado, Flaviano Godínez-Jaimes, Cruz Vargas-De-León, Norma Samanta Romero-Castro, Salvador Reyes-Fernández and Victor Othon Serna-Radilla

Abstract

Clinical designs in dentistry collect measurements of the teeth of each subject, forming complex data structures; however, standard statistical methods (Student's t-test, ANOVA, and regression models) do not treat the data as a grouped data type; that is, the measurements are treated as independent despite not being the case. A disadvantage of not considering the dependence on multilevel data is that if there is a significant correlation between the observations, it is ignored by the researcher and consequently finds statistically significant results when in fact they are not. Bayesian methods have the advantage of not assuming normality, unlike maximum likelihood estimation, and Bayesian methods are appropriate when you have small samples. We showed the minimum statistical theory for the use of multilevel models in dental research when the response variable is numerical. In this regard, it was proposed to carry out a Bayesian multilevel analysis to determine the clinical factors associated with the depth of periodontal probing. We adapted the bottom-up strategy to specify a multilevel model in the frequentist approach to the Bayesian approach. We checked the adequacy of the fit of the postulated model using posterior predictive density.

Keywords: periodontal probing depth, dental research, nested data structures, Bayesian multilevel modeling, bottom-up methodology

1. Introduction

The most widely used statistical methods in dental research are t-test, ANOVA (one, two and three factors), non-parametric tests, and regression models [1]. These methods assume that the observations of the studied variables are independent. Nested data structures are frequently found in dental research. An example is an experimental design in which multiple measurements are performed on the same individual. If, in addition to performing multiple measurements in an individual, we perform multiple measurements in each tooth, we will obtain a nested data structure. This nesting of the data results in grouped data. Typically, for clinical and dental data, contextual variables are measured in each individual (i.e., socioeconomic level, educational level, etc.), and these characteristics can form another group of data. Considering the detection of bacterial plaque in each tooth of individuals who have a home with a high marginality index, two nested groups are distinguished, namely, teeth nested in individuals and individuals nested at group. The word "nested" can be understood as "within" or "contained in." It is to be expected that items from the same group may be more similar to each other than items from a different group; that is, measurements from one individual are expected to be more similar to each other in comparison with measurements from other individuals. This fact indicates that the assumption of independence does not apply to nested data. Multilevel models take into account the non-independence of the observations. One consequence of ignoring the dependence of observations is that the results of some tests may be statistically significant when, actually, they are not. Under the classical approach, the estimation of the parameters of a multilevel model is performed using maximum likelihood, which has optimal properties in many scenarios; however, problems such as non-compliance with model assumptions or lack of convergence of iterative methods can occur. The Bayesian approach has some advantages over the classical approach.

The purpose of this chapter is to show the minimum statistical theory for the use of multilevel models in dental research when the response variable is numerical. For this, we will remember the definitions of multilevel models and multilevel generalized linear models (MGLM), in addition to the main Bayesian concepts and their application to MGLM. We will use an adaptation of the bottom-up strategy to specify a multilevel model. Our adaptation proposal tries to use the Bayesian leave-one-out cross-validation (LOO-CV) between the different steps for the comparison of models. We will check the adequacy of the fit of the postulated model using posterior predictive density. Finally, we will provide an example of this model applied to a numerical response variable, such as periodontal probing.

2. Multilevel models

Multilevel models partition the variance of the dependent variable at different levels of data grouping. At least two types of variance are distinguished: *intra-group variance* σ_w^2, or individual-level variance (level one), and *between-group variance* σ_b^2, which defines the variation at the group level (level two).

The dependency of the observations in the same group is measured with the *intraclass correlation coefficient* (ICC). Shrout and Fleiss in 1979 defined the ICC as the ratio of the *between-group variance* and the *total variance* (the sum of the variances between groups and in intra-groups):

$$ICC = \frac{\sigma_b^2}{\sigma_b^2 + \sigma_w^2} \tag{1}$$

The ICC varies between 0 and 1, since the variance cannot be negative. Before using a multilevel model, it is necessary to determine whether the ICC is significant at each level of the data. To that end, using the null model (defined in the next section), we determine whether the variance of the residuals of each level is significant. If that occurs, the ICC is also significant, and this means that at the individual level, the observations are dependent, and therefore, it is necessary to use a multilevel model instead of an ordinary multiple regression model [2].

2.1 Two-level models

Let y_{ij} be the dependent variable measured in the *i-th* individual in the *j-th* level-two unit (e.g., the j-th group); $i = 1, \dots, N$, where N is the total sample size, and $j = 1, \dots, J$ for J level-two units.

The simplest two-level model is the *null model (intercept-only model, unconditional means model, or one-way random-effects analysis of the variance)*. The model is defined by two equations:

$$\begin{aligned} y_{ij} &= \beta_{0j} + e_{ij} \\ \beta_{0j} &= \gamma_{00} + u_{0j} \end{aligned} \tag{2}$$

β_{0j} is the mean of y in the group j that varies across groups; e_{ij} is the individual variation around this mean; γ_{00} is the overall intercept, that is, the grand mean of y; and u_{0j} is the deviation of β_{0j} with respect to γ_{00}.

Substitution of β_{0j} in y_{ij} produces the single-equation model:

$$y_{ij} = \gamma_{00} + u_{0j} + e_{ij} \tag{3}$$

Eq. (3) is composed of a fixed part, γ_{00}, and a random part corresponding to two random effects, u_{0j} and e_{ij}. Assuming that $e_{ij} \sim N(0, \sigma^2)$ and $u_{0j} \sim N(0, \sigma^2_{u0})$ and that e_{ij} and u_{0j} are independent, the variance of y_{ij} in Eq. (3) is

$$\begin{aligned} var\left(y_{ij}\right) &= var\left(\gamma_{00} + u_{0j} + e_{ij}\right) \\ &= \sigma^2_{u0} + \sigma^2 \end{aligned} \tag{4}$$

where $\sigma^2_{u0} = \sigma^2_b$ is the variance between groups, and $\sigma^2 = \sigma^2_w$ is the variance within groups in Eq. (1) to calculate the ICC.

Now, let us consider a two-level model with two level-one independent variables, x_1 with a fixed effect α_1, which does not vary between groups, and x_2 with a random effect β_{2j}, which does vary between groups.

This model is defined by

$$\begin{aligned} y_{ij} &= \beta_{0j} + \alpha_1 x_{1ij} + \beta_{2j} x_{2ij} + e_{ij} \\ \beta_{0j} &= \gamma_{00} + \gamma_{01} w_{1j} + u_{0j} \\ \beta_{2j} &= \gamma_{10} + \gamma_{11} w_{1j} + u_{1j} \end{aligned} \tag{5}$$

In the above equation, both β_{0j} and β_{2j} depend on a level-two independent variable; w_1 and u_{qj} are the deviation of the effect of the variable w_1 on y_{ij} in the group j with respect to the average effect γ_{q0}.

Substitution of β_{0j} and β_{2j} in y_{ij} produces the single-equation model:

$$y_{ij} = \gamma_{00} + \alpha_1 x_{1ij} + \gamma_{01} w_{1j} + \gamma_{10} x_{2ij} + \gamma_{11} w_{1j} x_{2ij} + \left(u_{0j} + u_{1j} x_{2ij} + e_{ij}\right) \tag{6}$$

Generalizing the above two-level model to the case where level one includes P independent variables x_p that have a fixed effect, Q, independent variables x_q that have a random effect, and M level-two independent variables w_m, which also have a fixed effect, we have:

$$y_{ij} = \gamma_{00} + \sum_{m=1}^{M} \gamma_{0m} w_{mj} + \sum_{p=1}^{P} \alpha_p x_{pij} + \sum_{q=P+1}^{P+Q} \gamma_{q0} x_{qij} + \sum_{q=P+1}^{P+Q} \sum_{m=1}^{M} \gamma_{qm} w_{mj} x_{qij} + \left(u_{0j} + \sum_{q=P+1}^{P+Q} x_{qij} u_{qj} + e_{ij} \right) \quad (7)$$

Model 7 is composed of *fixed effects* (the coefficients γ and α) and *random effects* (all terms in parentheses). Two-level models can also be expressed in a matrix form by

$$Y = X\beta + Wu + e \quad (8)$$

where Y is the vector of measurements of the dependent variable, X is the design matrix of the fixed effect parameter vector β (containing the overall mean, main effects, and interactions), W is the design matrix of the random effects given by the vector U, and e is the vector of level-one residual errors.

2.2 Three-level models

Let i, j, and k indicate the observation units of levels 1, 2, and 3, respectively. In addition, level 3 has K units, each level-three unit has J_k level-two units, and the jth level-two unit in the kth level-three unit has n_{ijk} level-oneunits. The null model is

$$\begin{aligned} y_{ijk} &= \beta_{0jk} + e_{ijk} \\ \beta_{0jk} &= \gamma_{00k} + u_{0jk} \\ \gamma_{00k} &= \xi_{000} + \nu_{00k} \end{aligned} \quad (9)$$

In the first equation, β_{0jk} is the level-one random intercept that varies between the groups of level two, and e_{ijk} is the residual variance at level one with respect to β_{0jk}. In the second equation, γ_{00k} is the level-two random intercept that varies between the level-three units, and u_{0jk} is the residual variation of the group j with respect to γ_{00k}. In the third equation, ξ_{000} is the general intercept, that is, the grand mean of y, and ν_{00k} is the variation between the means of the level-three groups (i.e., the deviation of the mean of group k with respect to the grand mean).

Substituting γ_{00k} in β_{0jk} and then β_{0jk} in y_{ijk} yields

$$y_{ijk} = \xi_{000} + \nu_{00k} + u_{0jk} + e_{ijk} \quad (10)$$

Assuming that $e_{ijk} \sim N(0, \sigma^2)$, $u_{0jk} \sim N\left(0, \sigma^2_{u_0}\right)$, and $\nu_{00k} \sim N\left(0, \sigma^2_{\nu_0}\right)$ and that e_{ijk}, u_{0jk}, and ν_{00k} are independent, the variance of y_{ij} in Eq. (10) is

$$var\left(y_{ijk}\right) = \sigma^2_{\nu_0} + \sigma^2_{u0} + \sigma^2 \quad (11)$$

One way to define the ICC at levels two and three, attributed to Davis and Scott [3], is

$$\rho_{\text{level } 3} = \frac{\sigma^2_{\nu_0}}{\sigma^2_{\nu_0} + \sigma^2_{u_0} + \sigma^2} \quad (12)$$

$$\rho_{\text{level } 2} = \frac{\sigma^2_{u_0}}{\sigma^2_{\nu_0} + \sigma^2_{u_0} + \sigma^2}, \quad (13)$$

Now, we consider a three-level multilevel model with two level-one independent variables, x_1 and x_2; the former has a fixed effect and the latter a random effect:

$$y_{ijk} = \beta_{0jk} + \alpha_1 x_{1ijk} + \beta_{2jk} x_{2ijk} + e_{ijk} \tag{14}$$

Let suppose that the random coefficients β_{0jk} and β_{2jk} are explained by a second-level variable, w_1, by the relationships

$$\begin{aligned} \beta_{0jk} &= \gamma_{00k} + \gamma_{01k} w_{1jk} + u_{0jk} \\ \beta_{2jk} &= \gamma_{10k} + \gamma_{11k} w_{1jk} + u_{1jk} \end{aligned} \tag{15}$$

And the random coefficients in Eq. (15) are explained by a third-level variable, z_1, by the equations

$$\begin{aligned} \gamma_{00k} &= \xi_{000} + \xi_{001} z_{1k} + \nu_{00k} \\ \gamma_{01k} &= \xi_{010} + \xi_{011} z_{1k} + \nu_{01k} \\ \gamma_{10k} &= \xi_{100} + \xi_{101} z_{1k} + \nu_{10k} \\ \gamma_{11k} &= \xi_{110} + \xi_{111} z_{1k} + \nu_{11k} \end{aligned} \tag{16}$$

Substituting Eqs. (16) in (15) and then in Eq. (14), we have the three-level multilevel model:

$$\begin{aligned} y_{ijk} = {} & \xi_{000} + \alpha_1 x_{1ijk} + \xi_{001} z_{1k} + \xi_{010} w_{1jk} + \xi_{100} x_{2ijk} + \xi_{011} z_{1k} w_{1jk} \\ & + \xi_{101} z_{1k} x_{2ijk} + \xi_{110} w_{1jk} x_{2ijk} + \xi_{111} z_{1k} w_{1jk} x_{2ijk} \\ & + \left(u_{0jk} + \nu_{00k} + \nu_{10k} x_{2ijk} + u_{1jk} x_{2ijk} + \nu_{01k} w_{1jk} + \nu_{11k} w_{1jk} x_{2ijk} + e_{ijk} \right) \end{aligned} \tag{17}$$

where the regression coefficients ξ and α are the fixed part of the model, and the residual terms of each level contained in parentheses are the random part.

We can generalize the three-level model of Eq. (17). Suppose level one contains P independent variables x_p that have a fixed effect, α_p, and Q independent variables $x_q\, q = P+1, \dots, P+Q$. Level two contains M variables $w_m\, m = 1, \dots, M$. Level three contains L independent variables $z_l\, l = 1, \dots, L$.

$$\begin{aligned} y_{ijk} = {} & \xi_{000} + \sum_{p=1}^{P} \alpha_p x_{pijk} + \sum_{q=P+1}^{P+Q} \xi_{q00} x_{qijk} + \sum_{m=1}^{M} \xi_{0m0} w_{mjk} + \sum_{l=1}^{L} \xi_{00l} z_{lk} \\ & + \sum_{m=1}^{M} \sum_{l=1}^{L} \xi_{0ml} z_{lk} w_{mjk} + \sum_{q=P+1}^{P+Q} \sum_{l=1}^{L} \xi_{q0l} z_{lk} x_{qijk} + \sum_{q=P+1}^{P+Q} \sum_{m=1}^{M} \xi_{qm0} w_{mjk} x_{qijk} \\ & + \sum_{q=P+1}^{P+Q} \sum_{m=1}^{M} \sum_{l=1}^{L} \xi_{qml} z_{lk} w_{mjk} x_{qijk} + \left(\nu_{00k} + u_{0jk} + \sum_{q=P+1}^{P+Q} \nu_{10k} x_{qijk} \right. \\ & \left. + \sum_{q=P+1}^{P+Q} u_{qjk} x_{qijk} + \sum_{m=1}^{M} \nu_{0mk} w_{mjk} + \sum_{q=P+1}^{P+Q} \sum_{m=1}^{M} \nu_{qmk} w_{mjk} x_{qijk} + e_{ijk} \right). \end{aligned} \tag{18}$$

When the three-level model includes a random slope of level one and a random slope of level two, the model easily includes many parameters (interaction and a residual effect by each random slope coefficient) that easily cause convergence problems, except for sufficiently large data sets. Therefore, most three-level models have few random slope coefficients.

The equivalent matrix model for a three-level model is

$$Y = X\beta + Wu + Z\nu + e \tag{19}$$

Again, X is the design matrix of the fixed effect parameter vector β (containing the overall mean, main effects, and interactions), W is the design matrix of the random effects given by the vector u, Z is the design matrix of the random effects given by the vector ν, and e is the vector of level-one residual errors.

2.3 Assumptions of multilevel models

Statistical assumptions such as normal distribution, variance at each level, and independence between errors at different levels have been mentioned in the definition of the null multilevel model. They are explicitly defined in this section.

The dimension of the vector u depends on the number of random coefficients in the level-one equation; for example, in Eq. (14), the dimension is two. Similarly, the dimension of the vector ν depends on the number of random coefficients in the level-two equation; for example, in Eq. (15), the dimension is four. Let $e = (e_{111112}\cdots)^T$, $u = \left(u_{0jk}\, u_{1jk}\cdots u_{sjk}\right)^T$, and $\nu = (\nu_{00k}\cdots\nu_{0tk}\cdots\nu_{t0k}\cdots\nu_{ttk})^T$ with dimensions N, s, and t^2, respectively.

Multilevel models' assumptions are:

$$\begin{pmatrix} \nu \\ u \\ e \end{pmatrix} \sim N\left(\begin{pmatrix} \mathbf{0} \\ \mathbf{0} \\ \mathbf{0} \end{pmatrix}, \begin{pmatrix} D & \mathbf{0} & \mathbf{0} \\ \mathbf{0} & G & \mathbf{0} \\ \mathbf{0} & \mathbf{0} & R \end{pmatrix}\right) \tag{20}$$

where $\mathbf{0}$ is the vector of zeros with the appropriate dimension and

$$D = \begin{pmatrix} \sigma^2_{\nu 0} & \sigma_{\nu 01} & \cdots & \sigma_{\nu 0t} \\ \sigma_{\nu 01} & \sigma^2_{\nu 1} & \cdots & \sigma_{\nu 1t} \\ & \cdots & & \\ \sigma_{\nu 0t} & \sigma_{\nu 1t} & \cdots & \sigma^2_{\nu t} \end{pmatrix}, \quad G = \begin{pmatrix} \sigma^2_{u0} & \sigma_{u01} & \cdots & \sigma_{u0s} \\ \sigma_{u01} & \sigma^2_{u1} & \cdots & \sigma_{u1s} \\ & \cdots & & \\ \sigma_{u0s} & \sigma_{u1s} & \cdots & \sigma^2_{us} \end{pmatrix}, \quad R = \sigma^2 I \tag{21}$$

Eq. (20) says:

1. Level-one errors, e, are independent, identically normal distributed with mean zero and variance σ^2.

2. Level-two errors, u, follow a multivariate normal distribution with mean $\mathbf{0}$ and covariance G.

3. Level-three errors, ν, follow a multivariate normal distribution with mean $\mathbf{0}$ and covariance D.

4. Level-one and level-two errors are independent $Cov(e, u) = \mathbf{0}$.

5. Level-one and level-three errors are independent $Cov(e, \nu) = \mathbf{0}$.

6. Level-two and level-three errors are independent $Cov(u, \nu) = \mathbf{0}$.

2.4 Multilevel model estimation

The estimation of a multilevel model is complex because, in addition to the residuals at the individual level in the model, there are more residual terms of random intercepts and/or slopes of higher levels. Simultaneously, three types of parameters need to be estimated: the fixed effects, the random effects, and the residual variance/covariance components in matrices D, G, and R. Statistical theory and estimation algorithms for multilevel modeling are beyond the scope of this chapter, but some ideas are given.

When matrices D, G, and R are known, they can be used to estimate the combined model using generalized least square (GLS). The variance of y, given that the matrices D and G are known, is

$$\hat{V} = WDW' + ZGZ' + R \tag{22}$$

The inverse of the $\hat{V}$ matrix can be used as a weight; the regression coefficients of the model can be estimated using GLS. However, the matrices D and G are unknown.

The maximum likelihood estimation method is the most used for estimating multilevel models. It consists of maximizing the likelihood function that generally involves an iterative process that takes the parameter estimates as the initial parameter values for the next iteration of parameter estimation. This process is repeated until the parameter estimates have stabilized from one iteration to the next. The default *tolerance number*, which is sometimes defined by the users, is usually a sufficiently small number, for example, 10^{-8}. The model converges if the tolerance number is reached between two consecutive iterations. However, sometimes this does not happen. If the limit of specified iterations is reached and the tolerance number between two consecutive iterations has not been reached, the method is said to not converge, and this fact may indicate model specification problems or a small sample size.

Other estimation methods used in multilevel models are *generalized estimating equations*, *bootstrap methods,* and *Bayesian methods* [3]. When the assumptions of the multilevel models (Section 2.3) are not met, these methods are adequate.

2.5 Multilevel generalized linear models

Multilevel generalized linear models (MGLM) are an extension of generalized linear models. What makes both models different is that the former assumes dependence in the observations of the dependent variable and the latter assumes independence in the observations.

A three-level MGLM of the dependent variable Y conditioned in the random effects ν and u is

$$g[E(Y|\nu, \ u)] = \eta = X\beta + Wu + Z\nu \tag{23}$$

where $g(\cdot)$ is the link function, which is a known monotonic, differentiable function, and η is the linear predictor. As in multilevel models, the random effects are assumed to have a normal distribution with zero mean vector and variance/covariance matrixes D and G, respectively. The multilevel models described in Sections 2.1 and 2.2 are a particular case of MGLM with g, the identity function.

3. Bayesian inference

Bayesian inference is a more attractive alternative to frequentist maximum likelihood estimation when: (1) we have information about the parameters in the model, (2) the frequentist estimation method does not converge, (3) the sample size is small at the highest level of the data, or (4) nonlinear functions of the parameters are to be estimated. With this motivation, let us define some concepts.

The heart of the Bayesian inference is the posterior distribution of θ, $p(\theta|y)$, which is defined as the joint probability distribution of the observed data y and the parameter θ, $p(y,\theta) = p(y|\theta)p(\theta)$, conditioned on the known value of y, $p(y) = \int p(\theta)p(y|\theta)d\theta)$. Using Bayes' theorem, we obtain

$$p(\theta|y) = \frac{p(\theta)p(y|\theta)}{p(y)} \tag{24}$$

where $p(y|\theta)$ is the *likelihood* of the data y, and $p(\theta)$ is the *prior distribution* of $theta. p(y) = \int p(\theta)p(y|\theta)d\theta$ with fixed y is a normalization constant not depending on θ. So, an equivalent equation to (24) is

$$p(\theta|y) \propto p(\theta)p(y|\theta) \tag{25}$$

Prior distributions can be *informative* or *non-informative*. When the researcher has a high degree of certainty about θ, the prior distribution will have a small variance and so will also be informative. If this fact does not happen, that is, the researcher has low degree of certainty about θ, the prior distribution will have a large variance and so will be non-informative. Since the prior distribution is a factor in the posterior distribution, when the prior is informative, it will have a great impact on the posterior, so the researcher must be careful when an informative prior distribution is used.

Bayesian estimators are only mean or median vector of the posterior distribution, that is, $\hat{\theta} = \int \theta \frac{p(\theta)p(y|\theta)}{p(y)} d\theta$. However, if θ has high dimension, this implies to obtain multiple integrals that usually do not have a closed solution. Sometimes, $\theta = (\theta_a, \theta_b)$ and θ_b are nuisance parameters that must be ignored. The solution is to integrate the posterior distribution with respect to the nuisance parameters, but again, this multiple integral may have no closed solution.

The most widely used method is Markov chain Monte Carlo to obtain means, medians, and quantiles of the posterior distribution.

3.1 Markov chain Monte Carlo

3.1.1 Markov chain

A discrete-time *Markov chain* is a sequence of random variables, $X_n, n \geq 1$, that take values in a finite or countable Ω set that satisfies

$$p(X_{n+1} = j | X_0 = i_0, \ldots, X_n = i_n) = p(X_{n+1} = j | X_n = i_n) \tag{26}$$

for all n and any states $i_0, \ldots, i_n, j$ in Ω. Under regularity conditions, the chain will gradually forget its initial state i_0, and starting from a state t, $p^t(\cdot | X_0 = i_0)$ will converge to a unique stationary distribution $\phi(\cdot)$ (invariant) that does not depend on t or i_0.

As the number of sampled points $\{X_t\}$ increases, they will look more like dependent samples from $\phi(\cdot)$. The *burn-in* of an MCMC is the number of iterations, m, to eliminate so that the rest show a behavior of dependent samples from the stationary distribution $\phi(\cdot)$ [4]. When the number of burn-in samples is m, an estimator of the expectation of $f(X)$ is

$$E[\hat{f(X)}] = \frac{1}{n-m} \sum_{t=m+1}^{n} f(X_t) \tag{27}$$

3.1.2 Hamiltonian Monte Carlo

The Gibbs sampling and the random walk Metropolis are methods whose distributions converge to the target distributions; however, complex models with a large number of parameters may require an unacceptably long time to converge to the target distribution. This problem is largely caused by inefficient random walks that estimate the parameters' space.

The Hamiltonian Monte Carlo (HCM) algorithm or hybrid Monte Carlo algorithm eliminates random walks using momentum variables that transform the target distribution sampling problem into the Hamiltonian dynamics simulation problem. The Störmer–Verlet "leapfrog" (jump steps) integrator is used to simulate the time evolution of this system. Given a sample m, a step size ε, and a number of steps L, the HMC algorithm consists of resampling the momentum variables r_d from a standard multivariate normal distribution (it can be considered a Gibbs sampling update) and then applying L "leapfrog" updates to the position and momentum variables (θ and r) to generate a pair of proposed position and momentum variables ($\tilde{\theta}, \tilde{r}$), which are defined as $\theta^m = \tilde{\theta}$ and $r^m = \tilde{r}$, and will be accepted or rejected according to the Metropolis algorithm. For more details, see [5]. In general, specifying the step size (ε) and number of steps (L) is quite difficult when the path is too short, too long, or too straight.

This method for generating MCMC is implemented in the brms package [6] to perform Bayesian estimation in multilevel models.

3.1.3 MCMC diagnostics

After a large enough number of iterations, the MCMC eventually converges to the posterior distribution. A diagnostic statistic is needed to determine whether the MCMC has already converged to the stationary distribution or more iterations are needed. Several diagnostic statistics have been proposed, but we will use the Gelman and Rubin and graphical diagnostics.

Gelman and Rubin diagnostic *(GR)* [7]. This diagnostic uses several chains, $\{X_{i0}, \ldots, X_{in-1}\}$, $i = 1, \ldots, m$, drawn from an overdispersed density with respect to the target density $\pi(\cdot)$. In 1992, Gelman and Rubin defined two estimators of the variance of X when $X \sim \pi(\theta)$:

1. The *within-chain variance:* $W = \sum_{i=1}^{m}\sum_{j=0}^{n-1}\left(X_{ij} - \overline{X}_{i\cdot}\right)^2/(m(n-1))$ and

2. The *pooled variance:* $\hat{V} = ((n-1)/n)W + B/n.$

where $B/n = \sum_{i=1}^{m}\left(\overline{X}_{i\cdot} - \overline{X}_{\cdot\cdot}\right)^2/(m-1)$ is the *between-chain variance* estimate, $\overline{X}_{i\cdot}$ is the mean of the chain i, $i = 1, \ldots, m$, and $\overline{X}_{\cdot\cdot}$ is the overall mean. The potential scale reduction factor (PSRF) or Rhat is defined by:

$$\hat{R} = \frac{\hat{V}}{W} \tag{28}$$

The variance in the numerator of $\hat{R}$ overestimates the target variance, while the variance in the denominator underestimates it. This fact produces $\hat{R}$ greater than 1. One criterion for stopping the MCMC simulation is that $\hat{R} \approx 1$ or $\hat{R} < 1.1$. The GR and ESS diagnostics are implemented in the *coda* package [8].

Graphical diagnostics. MCMC trace plots are the most widely used diagnostic plots to determine convergence. They are a time series that shows the behavior of the Markov chains around their state space and their achievements at each iteration. When the visible trends show changes in the dispersion of the chain trace, the MCMC has not reached a stationary state. In contrast, when good mixing is observed, the MCMC sampling is said to converge to the target distribution.

3.2 Model checking and model comparison

Any Bayesian analysis should include a check of the adequacy of the fit of the postulated model to the data. The adequacy of the fit of a model is measured by how well the distribution of the proposed model approximates the distribution of the data; the better the fit of the postulated model to the data, the better the model. But if the fit is poor, it does not mean that the model is bad, but rather that it contains deficiencies that can be improved. This section explains a model assessment method based on the posterior predictive distribution.

Let us define the replicated data y^{rep} as one that could be observed tomorrow if the experiment that produced the current data y were replicated tomorrow with the same model and the same values of θ that produced y. The distribution of y^{rep} given the current data y is called *posterior predictive distribution* and defined as [9].

$$p(y^{rep}|y) = \int p(y^{rep}|\theta)p(\theta|y)d\theta \tag{29}$$

If the model is accurate, that is, it has a reasonably good fit, the replicated data should be similar to the observed data.

3.2.1 Log pointwise predictive density

The performance of the fitted model can be measured by the quality of its predictions in the new data y^f. Pointwise predictions are predictions of each element y_i^f in y^f that are summarized using an appropriate statistic.

Access to y^f is not always easy and sometimes impossible. Instead, performance of the fitted model can be done using the current data y. This method for calculating predictive accuracy and to compare models is known as *within-sample predictive accuracy*.

The *log pointwise predictive density* (lppd) of the fitted model to the observed data and unknown parameter θ is defined as

$$lppd = \log \prod_{i=1}^{n} p(\theta|y_i) = \sum_{i=1}^{n} \log \int p(y_i|\theta)p(\theta|y_i)d\theta \tag{30}$$

In general, the expected predictive accuracy of a model fitted to new data is poorer than the expected predictive accuracy of the same model with the observed data. With the *computed lppd* (clppd), we can evaluate the expression using draws from $p(\theta|y)$ obtained with MCMC, θ^s, $s = 1, \dots, S$ using sufficient draws:

$$clppd = \sum_{i=1}^{n} \log \left(\frac{1}{S} \sum_{s=1}^{S} p(y_i|\theta^s) \right) \tag{31}$$

The clppd of the observed data y is an overestimate of the clppd for future data.

A second method to assess posterior predictive expectation is the *adjusted within-sample predictive accuracy* that consists of a bias correction of the lppd estimated using information criteria such as Akaike information criterion, deviance information criterion, or Watanabe–Akaike information criterion.

A third method to assess posterior predictive expectation is the *cross-validation*, which captures the out-of-sample predictive error by fitting the model to the training data and assessing the predictive fit in the holdout data [9]. In model comparison, the best model is the one with the lowest predictive error. Let us explain this method in detail:

Leave-one-out cross-validation (LOO-CV) works with n partitions in which each holdout set has only one observation, which generates n different inferences, $p_{post(-i)}$, obtained through S posterior simulations, θ^{is}.

The Bayesian LOO-CV estimate of the predictive fit out of the sample is

$$lppd_{loo-cv} = \sum_{i=1}^{n} \log p_{post(-i)}(y_i) \approx \sum_{i=1}^{n} \log \left(\frac{1}{S} \sum_{s=1}^{S} p(y_i|\theta^{is}) \right) \tag{32}$$

Each prediction is conditioned in $n - 1$ data points, which underestimates the predictive fit. For large n, the difference is insignificant; however, for small n, a first-order bias correction $b = lppd - \overline{lppd}_{-i}$ can be used, where

$$\overline{lppd}_{-i} = \frac{1}{n} \sum_{i=1}^{n} \sum_{j=1}^{n} \log p_{post(-i)}(y_j) \approx \frac{1}{n} \sum_{i=1}^{n} \sum_{j=1}^{n} \log \left(\frac{1}{S} \sum_{s=1}^{S} p(y_j|\theta^{is}) \right) \tag{33}$$

The bias-corrected Bayesian LOO-CV is

$$lppd_{cloo-cv} = lppd_{loo-cv} + b \tag{34}$$

An estimation of the effective number of parameters is

$$p_{loo-cv} = ldpp - ldpp_{loo-cv} \tag{35}$$

When comparing two fitted models, we can estimate the difference in their expected predictive accuracy by the difference in $elppd_{loo-cv}$. The standard error of the difference can be computed using a paired estimate to take advantage of the fact that the same set of n data points is used to fit both models.

Suppose we are comparing models I and II, with corresponding fit measures $elpd^{I}_{loo-cv}$ and $elpd^{II}_{loo-cv}$; then difference and its standard error are

$$\begin{aligned} elpd\_diff &= elpd^{I}_{loo-cv} - elpd^{II}_{loo-cv} \\ se\_diff &= se\left(elpd^{I}_{loo-cv} - elpd^{II}_{loo-cv}\right) = \sqrt{nV^{n}_{i}\left(elpd^{I}_{loo,i} - elpd^{II}_{loo,i}\right)} \end{aligned} \tag{36}$$

When two models are compared using the LOO-CV statistic, the one with the lowest value of this statistic is declared the best model. If elpd_diff is used with the loo_compare function of the brms library [6], the value of the difference is reported in the best model accompanied by its se_diff. When comparing two models, the value of the difference is reported in the column of the best model. There is more evidence of the superiority of one model over another when the elpd_diff is larger than the se_diff.

4. Multilevel model methodology

To propose a multilevel model, it is necessary to determine which variables will be in the fixed part, which in the random part, and the cross-level interactions. This task can be complex, so we need a strategy to build the model.

4.1 Multilevel model building strategy

In this section, we show an adaptation of the bottom-up strategy to specify a three-level multilevel model. The bottom-up methodology is used in the frequentist approach [3]. Our adaptation proposal tries to use the Bayesian LOO-CV from Step 2 to Step 7 for model comparison.

Step 1. Fitting the intercept-only model:

$$y_{ijk} = \xi_{000} + \left(\nu_{00k} + u_{0jk} + e_{ijk}\right) \tag{37}$$

This model gives a basal line to compare with the next models.

Step 2. Add all the level-one independent variables fixed:

$$y_{ijk} = \xi_{000} + \sum_{p=1}^{P} \alpha_p x_{pijk} + \sum_{q=P+1}^{P+Q} \xi_{q00} x_{qijk} + \left(\nu_{00k} + u_{0jk} + e_{ijk}\right) \tag{38}$$

It must be determined which level-one variable has a significant effect on y. We will assume that all the P level-one variables are statistically significant. Models 38 and 37 must be compared.

Step 3. Add the level-two independent variables fixed:

$$y_{ijk} = \xi_{000} + \sum_{p=1}^{P} \alpha_p x_{pijk} + \sum_{q=P+1}^{P+Q} \xi_{q00} x_{qijk} + \sum_{m=1}^{M} \xi_{0m0} w_{mjk} + \left(\nu_{00k} + u_{0jk} + e_{ijk}\right) \tag{39}$$

It must be determined which level-two variable has a significant effect on y. If the variables w_m explain the variability of y, Model 39 should be superior to Model 38. Again, we assume that all the M level-two independent variables are statistically significant.

Step 4. Add the level-three independent variables fixed:

$$\begin{aligned} y_{ijk} = {} & \xi_{000} + \sum_{p=1}^{P} \alpha_p x_{pijk} + \sum_{q=P+1}^{P+Q} \xi_{q00} x_{qijk} + \sum_{m=1}^{M} \xi_{0m0} w_{mjk} + \sum_{l=1}^{L} \xi_{00l} z_{lk} \\ & + \left(\nu_{00k} + u_{0jk} + e_{ijk}\right) \end{aligned} \tag{40}$$

It must be determined which level-three variable has a significant effect on y. If the variables z_l explain the variability of y, Model 40 should be superior to Model 39.

Steps 1–3 consider the specification of the fixed part of the three-level multilevel model. Now we will specify the random part of the model.

Step 5. Assessing whether any of the slopes of the independent variables at level one has a significative variance component between groups at level two or level three.

$$\begin{aligned} y_{ijk} = {} & \xi_{000} + \sum_{p=1}^{P} \alpha_p x_{pijk} + \sum_{q=P+1}^{P+Q} \xi_{q00} x_{qijk} + \sum_{m=1}^{M} \xi_{0m0} w_{mjk} + \sum_{l=1}^{L} \xi_{00l} z_{lk} \\ & + \left(\nu_{00k} + u_{0jk} + \sum_{q=P+1}^{P+Q} \nu_{q0k} x_{qijk} + \sum_{q=P+1}^{P+Q} u_{qjk} x_{qijk} + e_{ijk}\right) \end{aligned} \tag{41}$$

where u_{qjk} are the level-two residuals of the slopes of the level-one independent variable x_q, and ν's are the level-three residuals of the slopes of the level-two independent variable w_m.

Level-one independent variables that do not have a significant slope may have a significant random slope. This step and the next should be carefully performed, because the model can easily become overparameterized and/or have problems such as non-convergence or extremely slow calculations. It is advisable to assess significance of the slopes variable by variable. Next, the model is formulated with all the variables with significant random slopes. If Model 41 is not better than Model 40, the procedure for specifying a three-level multilevel model stops.

Step 6. Assessing whether any of the slopes of the level-two independent variable has a significant variance component among level-three groups.

$$\begin{aligned} y_{ijk} = {} & \xi_{000} + \sum_{p=1}^{P} \alpha_p x_{pijk} + \sum_{q=P+1}^{P+Q} \xi_{q00} x_{qijk} + \sum_{m=1}^{M} \xi_{0m0} w_{mjk} + \sum_{l=1}^{L} \xi_{00l} z_{lk} \\ & + \left(\nu_{00k} + u_{0jk} + \sum_{q=P+1}^{P+Q} \nu_{q0k} x_{qijk} + \sum_{q=P+1}^{P+Q} u_{qjk} x_{qijk} + \sum_{m=1}^{M} \nu_{0mk} w_{mjk} + e_{ijk}\right) \end{aligned} \tag{42}$$

where the ν's are the level-three residuals of the slopes of the level-two independent variable w_m.

The assessment of random slopes of the level-two variables should be performed variable by variable, and then, all these variables should be included into a model to assess the improvement of the model with respect to Model 41.

Step 7. Adding interactions between level-three independent variables and the level-one and level-two independent variables that have a significant slope variance in Steps 5 and 6. This produces the full model:

$$\begin{aligned} y_{ijk} = {} & \xi_{000} + \sum_{p=1}^{P} \alpha_p x_{pijk} + \sum_{q=P+1}^{P+Q} \xi_{q00} x_{qijk} + \sum_{m=1}^{M} \xi_{0m0} w_{mjk} + \sum_{l=1}^{L} \xi_{00l} z_{lk} \\ & + \sum_{m=1}^{M} \sum_{l=1}^{L} \xi_{0ml} z_{lk} w_{mjk} + \sum_{q=P+1}^{P+Q} \sum_{l=1}^{L} \xi_{q0l} z_{lk} x_{qijk} + \sum_{q=P+1}^{P+Q} \sum_{m=1}^{M} \xi_{qm0} w_{mjk} x_{qijk} \\ & + \sum_{q=P+1}^{P+Q} \sum_{m=1}^{M} \sum_{l=1}^{L} \xi_{qml} z_{lk} w_{mjk} x_{qijk} + \left(\nu_{00k} + u_{0jk} + \sum_{q=P+1}^{P+Q} \nu_{q0k} x_{qijk} \right. \\ & \left. + \sum_{q=P+1}^{P+Q} u_{qjk} x_{qijk} + \sum_{m=1}^{M} \nu_{0mk} w_{mjk} + \sum_{q=P+1}^{P+Q} \sum_{m=1}^{M} \nu_{qmk} w_{mjk} x_{qijk} + e_{ijk} \right). \end{aligned} \tag{43}$$

When explaining the variances of the random slopes in terms of contextual variables, the model automatically includes interaction terms between levels that compose the fixed part of the model. It is recommended to add variables that explain the variance of the random slope coefficients one by one and not as shown in this step (this was done here to avoid specifying more equations).

When it comes to an MGLM, the methodology changes slightly; that is, instead of defining models in terms of y, models are defined in terms of $g\left(\mu_{ijk}\right) = g\left(E\left[Y_{ijk} | \nu, u\right]\right)$, and the residual errors at the individual level are no longer specified. An example of this methodology for an MGLM is illustrated below.

5. Application: periodontal probing depth

In this section, an example is given in which a multilevel generalized linear model is used for data from a cross-sectional study conducted by Romero-Castro et al. [10]. This study was carried out among adults who reside in the state of Guerrero, Mexico, and who went to the external dental clinical service of the Dental School of the Autonomous University of Guerrero (UAGro) in search of treatment, during the period from August 2015 to February 2016. The protocol was approved (registration no. CB005/2015) by the ethic committee at UAGro.

The goal of this multilevel analysis was to determine the clinical factors associated with the depth of periodontal probing.

Thirty-two teeth were examined in each of the 116 patients. Probing pocket depth was recorded at six sites in each tooth, that is, *mesiobuccal, mid buccal, distobuccal, mesiolingual, mid lingual,* and *distolingual* locations of each tooth. Pocket depth was recorded by use of Florida probe in the six sites. The response variable was *probing depth* measured in millimeters; that is, probing depth is a continuous variable and greater than zero (≥ 0). The data set consisted of 18,358 observations.

The independent variables, except the age, were all dichotomous: *bleeding, mobility, plaque, calculus, insulin resistance (fasting plasma glucose* $> 100\ mg/dL$*), smoking, root remnants, and mismatched restorations*, where 0 indicated absence and 1 presence.

Figure 1 and **Table 1** show the three levels of the data and the variables at each level. The first level corresponded to the probing sites where the independent variables *bleeding* and *furcation* and the response variable *probing depth* were measured. Level two corresponded to the dental piece, that is, teeth that only had the independent variable *mobility*, and level three corresponded to the patients, measuring the independent variables *age, plaque, calculus, insulin resistance, smoking, root remnants*, and *mismatched restorations*.

A first data analysis was done using a three-level multilevel model assuming a normal distribution for the probing depth. The frequentist fit had two problems: the residuals did not have a normal distribution and the numerical method to obtain the estimates did not converge.

The minimum of probing depth was 0.2 mm, Q1 was 0.8 mm, Q2 was 1.2 mm, Q3 was 1.8 and the maximum was 9 mm. In addition, its distribution was asymmetric to the right (skewness = 1.6 and kurtosis = 8.0). Therefore, it was assumed that probing depth had gamma distribution with mean μ and variance μ^2/α:

$$f(y) = \frac{(\alpha/\mu)^{\alpha}}{\Gamma(\alpha)} y^{\alpha-1} \exp\left(-\frac{\alpha y}{\mu}\right) \tag{44}$$

It is well known that gamma regression belongs to the generalized linear model family. But as the data studied is of hierarchical nature, the appropriate model is the

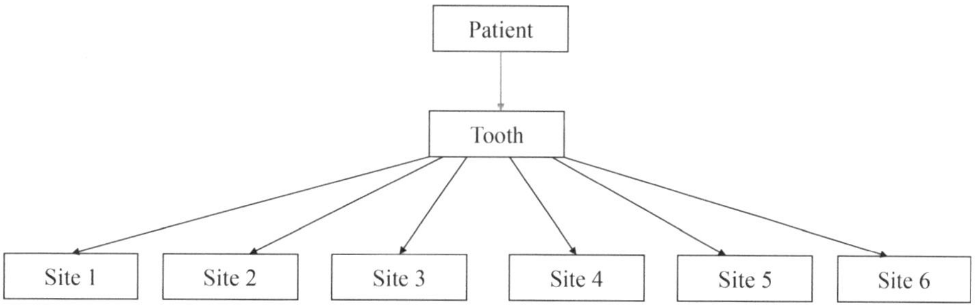

Figure 1.
Multilevel structure of the probing depth of 1 tooth out of 32 teeth for each patient.

Levels	Variables
Level 3: Patient	Age, plaque, calculus, insulin resistance, smoke, root remnants, and mismatched restorations
Level 2: Tooth	Mobility
Level 1: Probing site	Bleeding

Table 1.
Independent variables on levels.

multilevel generalized linear model. Given that the response variable is non-negative, the link function used was the natural logarithm to get expected probing depth greater than zero.

5.1 Bayesian estimation

Likelihood: It was assumed that probing depth follows a gamma distribution.

Prior distribution: It was defined as a product of marginal prior distributions for each component of β in Model 23. β is composed by the overall mean, main effects, and interactions: $\xi_{000}, \xi_{q00}, \xi_{0m0}, \xi_{00l}, \xi_{0ml}, \xi_{q0l}, \xi_{qm0}, \xi_{qml}$, and all of them had $N(0, 10^2)$ prior. *brms* function uses a special parameterization for matrices D and G in Eq. (21). This parameterization is $G = F(\sigma_k)\Omega_k F(\sigma_k)$, where $F(\sigma_k)$ is a diagonal matrix with diagonal elements σ_k [6]. Priors for D and G needed only to specify priors for σ_k and Ω_k, which were $\sigma_k \sim HalfCauchy(10)$ and $\Omega_k \sim CorrLKJ(1)$. Finally, the shape hyper-parameter was $shape \sim \mathcal{G}amma(0.01{,}0.01)$.

The analysis of this model was performed with the *brms* library [6, 11] that uses the probabilistic programming language *Stan* [12] in the environment of *R Software 4.0.5*.

Simulation: All the MCMC had four chains; the number of iterations and burn-in was not the same for the models studied, but all used a final sample of 4000.

The MCMC of the models (37, 38 and 39), that is, null, with level-one, and with level-two variables, were obtained using 4000 iterations and a burn-in of 3000. Model 40 used 5000 iterations and a burn-in of 4000, Model 41 used 7000 iterations and a burn-in of 6000, and Model 43 used 8000 iterations and a burn-in of 7000.

Bayesian estimators: The mean of the posterior distribution was used as the Bayesian estimator; this is related with minimizing the squared loss function.

Models studied: We studied a three-level multilevel generalized linear model, where i represented the level-one units, j the level-two units, and k the level-three units. Although the values of the Rhats are not shown, all the MCMC of the studied models converged since all the Rhats were at most 1.01.

Step 1. The null model is

$$log\left(\mu_{ijk}\right) = \xi_{000} + \left(\nu_{00k} + u_{0jk}\right) \tag{45}$$

Columns 2 and 3 of **Table 2** show the Bayesian estimations of the null model. The credible intervals did not contain zero, so that the variances at the tooth level and at the patient level were significant. This supports the use of MGLM.

Step 2. The model with level-one variable, *bleeding*, is

$$log\left(\mu_{ijk}\right) = \xi_{000} + \alpha_1 \text{bleeding}_{1ijk} + \left(\nu_{00k} + u_{0jk}\right) \tag{46}$$

The Bayesian estimations of the model showed that the bleeding coefficient was significant (columns 4 and 5 of **Table 2**). The comparison of Models 45 and 46, using LOO-CV, indicates that the model including the level-one variables was better (before the last row and column 5 in **Table 2**).

Step 3. The model with level-two variable, *mobility*, is

$$log\left(\mu_{ijk}\right) = \xi_{000} + \alpha_1 \text{bleeding}_{1ijk} + \xi_{010} \text{mobility}_{1jk} + \left(\nu_{00k} + u_{0jk}\right) \tag{47}$$

DOI: http://dx.doi.org/10.5772/intechopen.108442

	Model 45		Model 46		Model 47		Model 48		Model 49		Model 50	
	Coef	**(95%CrI)**	**Coef**	**(95%CrI)**	**Coef**	**(95%CrI)**	**Coef**	**(95%CrI)**	**Coef**	**(95%CrI)**	**Coef**	**(95%CrI)**
Group-level effects:												
Patient (116 levels)												
sd(Intercept)	0.20	(0.17, 0.23)	0.20	(0.17, 0.23)	0.20	(0.17, 0.23)	0.19	(0.17, 0.22)	0.19	(0.17, 0.22)	0.19	(0.17, 0.22)
sd(Bleeding)									0.12	(0.02, 0.21)	0.13	(0.02, 0.23)
Patient:Tooth (3131 levels)												
sd(Intercept)	0.23	(0.22, 0.24)	0.22	(0.21, 0.23)	0.22	(0.21, 0.23)	0.22	(0.21, 0.23)	0.22	(0.21, 0.23)	0.22	(0.21, 0.23)
sd(Bleeding)									0.25	(0.16, 0.33)	0.25	(0.16, 0.34)
Population-level effects:												
Intercept	0.34	(0.30, 0.37)	0.33	(0.29, 0.37)	0.33	(0.29, 0.36)	0.29	(0.24, 0.34)	0.29	(0.25, 0.34)	0.29	(0.25, 0.34)
Bleeding			0.15	(0.11, 0.19)	0.15	(0.10, 0.19)	0.15	(0.10, 0.19)	0.13	(0.07, 0.20)	0.11	(0.02, 0.19)
Mobility					0.04	(−0.00, 0.08)	0.03	(−0.01, 0.07)	0.03	(−0.01, 0.07)	0.03	(−0.01, 0.08)
Calculus							0.10	(0.03, 0.18)	0.10	(0.03, 0.18)	0.10	(0.03, 0.18)
Smoking							−0.02	(−0.14, 0.09)	−0.02	(−0.14, 0.10)	−0.02	(−0.13, 0.09)
Bleeding:Calculus											0.06	(−0.07, 0.19)
Specific parameters:												
Shape	4.50	(4.41, 4.60)	4.51	(4.41, 4.61)	4.51	(4.41.4.61)	4.51	(4.42, 4.61)	4.55	(4.45, 4.64)	4.54	(4.45, 4.64)
elpd_diff (se_diff)				−16.2 (8.2)†		−2.3 (2.0)‡		−3.4 (1.5)◆		−10.7 (7.9)#		−1.3 (1.8)*

Coef: Coefficient.
**95%CrI: 95% Credible Interval. Comparisons.†Model 45 vs. 46.‡Model 46 vs. 47. Model 47 vs. 48.#Model 48 vs. 49.*Model 49 vs. 50.*

Table 2.
Bayesian estimates of Models 45–50.

Mobility fixed effect was not significant (columns 6 and 7 of **Table 2**); however, it was retained in the model because it was the only level-two variable and to get estimations of the effect of the third-level independent variables adjusted for the effect of level-two variable. The LOO-CV criterion indicated that this model was slightly better (before the last row and column 7 in **Table 2**).

There are seven level-three contextual variables (**Table 1**); before specifying the model containing only the significant level-three variables, a forward selection of variables was performed to avoid having an overparameterized model. **Table 3** shows the variable selection procedure where each model contains the level-one variable, *bleeding*, and the level-two variable, *mobility*. The LOO-CV model comparison indicates that the model that includes *calculus* and *smoking* variables is the best model.

Step 4. The model with level-three variables, *calculus* and *smoking*, is

$$\begin{aligned} log\left(\mu_{ij|k}\right) &= \xi_{000} + \alpha_1 \text{bleeding}_{1ijk} + \xi_{010}\text{mobility}_{1jk} \\ &+ \xi_{001}\text{calculus}_{1k} + \xi_{002}\text{smoking}_{2k} + \left(\nu_{00k} + u_{0jk}\right) \end{aligned} \tag{48}$$

Columns 8 and 9 in **Table 2** show that the variable *smoking* was not significant; however, the model that contains smoking is better than the others. Model 48 was better than Model 47 (before the last row and column 9 in **Table 2**).

Step 5. The model with a random slope for the variable bleeding.

In Eq. (49), a random slope for the variable bleeding is added that varies at patient and teeth levels; that is, the relationship between probing depth and bleeding varied between patients and between teeth.

$$\begin{aligned} log\left(\mu_{ij|k}\right) &= \xi_{000} + \alpha_1 \text{bleeding}_{1ijk} + \xi_{010}\text{mobility}_{1jk} \\ &+ \xi_{001}\text{calculus}_{1k} + \xi_{002}\text{smoking}_{2k} \\ &+ \nu_{10k}\text{bleeding}_{1ijk} + u_{1jk}\text{bleeding}_{1ijk} + \left(\nu_{00k} + u_{0jk}\right) \end{aligned} \tag{49}$$

Finally, in the next model interaction, terms were added based on signs that occur in periodontal disease.

Columns 10 and 11 of **Table 2** show that the random slope of bleeding was significant at patient and teeth levels. Again, this model was compared with Model 48 using the LOO-CV criterion, and the best model was Model 48, which contained random slopes (before the last row and column 11 in **Table 2**).

Step 7. The model with cross-level interactions is

$$\begin{aligned} log\left(\mu_{ij|k}\right) &= \xi_{000} + \alpha_1 \text{bleeding}_{1ijk} + \xi_{010}\text{mobility}_{1jk} \\ &+ \xi_{001}\text{calculus}_{1k} + \xi_{002}\text{smoking}_{2k} + \xi_{101}\text{bleeding}_{1ijk}\text{calculus}_{1k} \\ &+ \nu_{10k}\text{bleeding}_{1ijk} + u_{1jk}\text{bleeding}_{1ijk} + \left(\nu_{00k} + u_{0jk}\right) \end{aligned} \tag{50}$$

Eq. (50) has an interaction between the level-three variable calculus with the level-one variable bleeding. Columns 12 and 13 of **Table 2** show that the interaction was not significant (its credible interval contained zero). Finally, the comparison of models indicated that the best model was Model 49 corresponding to the bleeding random slope model (the last row and column 13 in **Table 2**). So, this model is interpreted.

Figure 2 shows the posterior predictive fit of Model 49 to the data. The replicated data are plotted in a light color, and the observed data are plotted in black. As both

Model	elpd_diff	se_diff
Comparison of models with one level-three independent variable.		
$\xi_{001}\text{calculus}_{1k}$	0.0	0.0
$\xi_{003}\text{insulin resistance}_{3k}$	−0.1	1.6
$\xi_{004}\text{root remnants}_{4k}$	−0.8	1.5
$\xi_{005}\text{plaque}_{5k}$	−1.5	1.6
$\xi_{002}\text{smoking}_{2k}$	−1.7	1.6
$\xi_{006}\text{age}_{6k}$	−1.8	1.5
$\xi_{007}\text{mismatched restorations}_{7k}$	−2.5	1.5
Comparison of models with two level-three independent variables.		
$\xi_{001}\text{calculus}_{1k} + \xi_{002}\text{smoking}_{2k}$	0.0	0.0
$\xi_{001}\text{calculus}_{1k} + \xi_{003}\text{insulin resistance}_{3k}$	−2.1	1.5
$\xi_{001}\text{calculus}_{1k} + \xi_{006}\text{age}_{6k}$	−2.6	1.5
$\xi_{001}\text{calculus}_{1k} + \xi_{005}\text{plaque}_{5k}$	−2.9	1.5
$\xi_{001}\text{calculus}_{1k} + \xi_{007}\text{mismatched restorations}_{7k}$	−4.4	1.5
$\xi_{001}\text{calculus}_{1k} + \xi_{004}\text{root remnants}_{4k}$	−5.2	1.5
Comparison of the best models with one and two level-three independent variables		
$\xi_{001}\text{calculus}_{1k} + \xi_{002}\text{smoking}_{2k}$	0.0	0.0
$\xi_{001}\text{calculus}_{1k}$	−2.6	1.5
Comparison of models with three level-three independent variables		
$\xi_{001}\text{calculus}_{1k} + \xi_{002}\text{smoking}_{2k} + \xi_{004}\text{rootremnants}_{4k}$	0.0	0.0
$\xi_{001}\text{calculus}_{1k} + \xi_{002}\text{smoking}_{2k} + \xi_{006}\text{age}_{6k}$	−0.2	1.6
$\xi_{001}\text{calculus}_{1k} + \xi_{002}\text{smoking}_{2k} + \xi_{003}\text{insulin resistance}_{3k}$	−0.6	1.5
$\xi_{001}\text{calculus}_{1k} + \xi_{002}\text{smoking}_{2k} + \xi_{005}\text{plaque}_{5k}$	−1.2	1.6
$\xi_{001}\text{calculus}_{1k} + \xi_{002}\text{smoking}_{2k} + \xi_{007}\text{mismatchedrestorations}_{7k}$	−1.6	1.5
Comparison of the best models with two and three level-three independent variables		
$\xi_{001}\text{calculus}_{1k} + \xi_{002}\text{smoking}_{2k}$	0.0	0.0
$\xi_{001}\text{calculus}_{1k} + \xi_{002}\text{smoking}_{2k} + \xi_{004}\text{root remnants}_{4k}$	−2.9	1.5

[*] *All the models have the structure:* $\log\left(\mu_{ij|k}\right) = \xi_{000} + \alpha_1\text{bleeding}_{1ijk} + \xi_{010}\text{mobility}_{1jk} + \text{var1} + \text{var2} + \text{var3} + (\nu_{00k} + u_{0jk})$, *where* var1 *is the independent variable that produces the best fit among all the seven models with one independent variable. Similarly,* var2 *is the second independent variable that produces the best fit among all the six models, having* var1 *in common, with two independent variables, and so on for* var3.

Table 3.
Forward variable selection for the level-three variables[*].

curves agree very well, the posterior predictive density fits very well with the distribution of the probing depth. Both distributions are clearly not symmetric, and they seem to follow a gamma distribution. Definitely, normal distribution was not an appropriate assumption for probing depth. In conclusion, the random slope model (49) had a good fit.

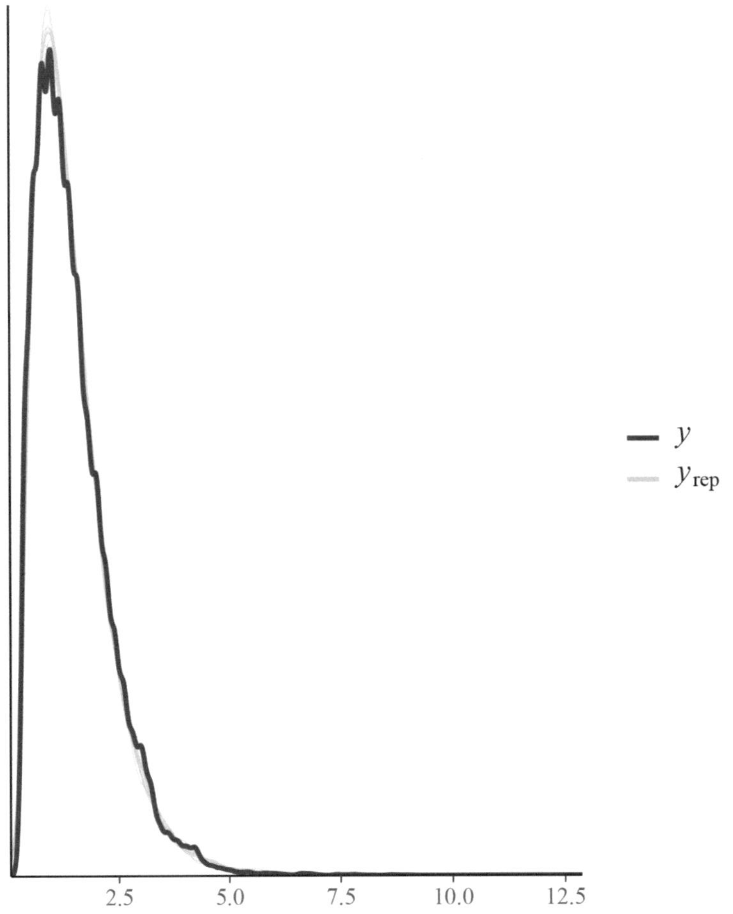

Figure 2.
Posterior predictive density of Model 49 with a random slope for bleeding between teeth and patient.

Figure 3 shows the histograms of the empirical posterior distributions of the parameters. Finally, the MCMC of Model 49 converged since all the Rhats were at most 1.01, and the trace plots of **Figure 3** show that the chains mix well.

5.2 Discussion

In this example of probing depth, the variance at the tooth level (1.59) and the variance at the patient level (1.49) were significant (**Table 2**); that is, the mean of the dependent variable varied between teeth nested in patients, and the ICC at the tooth level (0.45) was higher than that at the patient level (0.42); that is, there was greater dependence between the measurements of the probing sites of different teeth than between measurements of the probing sites of different patients. This finding probes that using a multilevel model for these probing depth data was better than using a single-level model, and the former produced more accurate estimates and credible intervals. In addition, the random slope of bleeding was significant between teeth; that is, there was a positive relationship between probing depth and bleeding that varied between teeth in the patients (probing depth between teeth increased by an average of 1.28 mm if the site was bleeding). On the other hand,

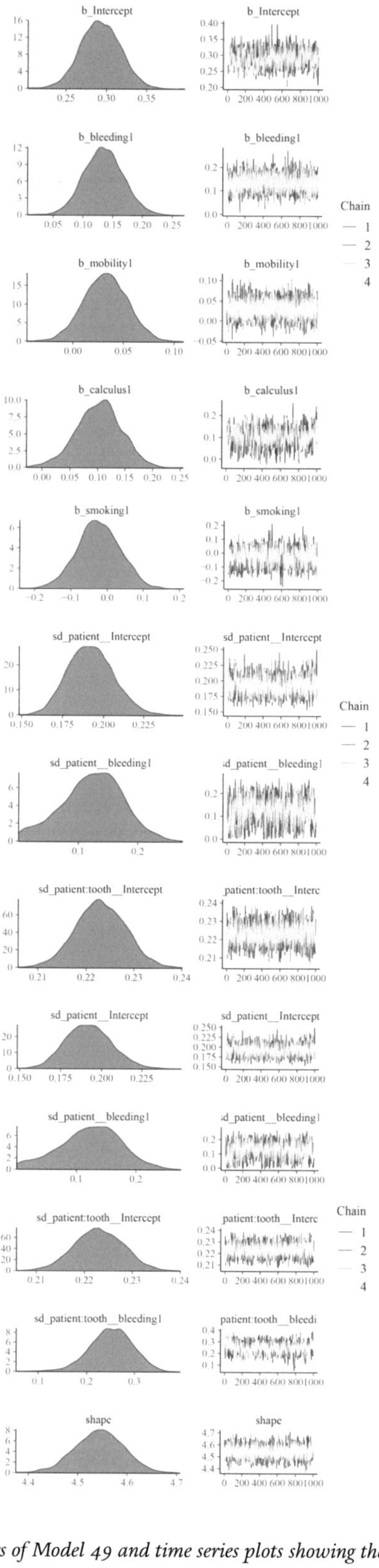

Figure 3.
Posterior distribution of parameters of Model 49 and time series plots showing the MCMC output.

calculus is a form of hardened dental plaque. In the random slope model (Eq. (49)), bleeding and calculus were significant parameters that estimated that, on average, the depth of bleeding probing sites was 1.14 mm greater than the sites that did not exhibit bleeding. On average, the probing depth of patients who had calculus on any of the teeth was 1.11 mm greater than of patients who did not have calculus. The plausible intervals for bleeding and calculus were (1.07,1.22) and (1.03,1.20), respectively.

In the random slope model, mobility and smoking were not significantly associated with probing depth, but if we decide to give them an interpretation, we can say that, on average, the probing depth of patients who presented dental mobility was 1.03 mm greater than the probing depth of patients who did not have dental mobility. Similarly, smoking patients had, on average, a probing depth 0.98 mm greater than that in non-smoking patients. Different results and interpretations could be obtained from measuring the independent variables at levels other than those given in this example. Specifically, the variable calculus could have been measured at the tooth level. Before fitting the Bayesian multilevel model, we tried to estimate the multilevel model using restricted maximum likelihood; however, the numerical method did not converge. More practical examples using the *R Software* can be found at [13].

6. Conclusions

In certain clinical research designs, the data have a nested structure (in other words, a hierarchical structure). The data that make up a nested structure are modeled using multilevel models because they simultaneously estimate the effects of the variables at the individual level and the effects of the contextual variables or variables at the group level. A significant ICC determines whether it is necessary to use a multilevel model. If the ICC is not significant, an ordinary regression model is sufficient to model the nested data. A disadvantage of multilevel models is that they easily contain a large number of parameters to be estimated. On the other hand, modeling the data levels separately incurs a large type 1 error even when the ICC is small. This fact causes the inferences to be incorrect. The maximum likelihood estimation of the parameters of a multilevel model requires that the assumptions of the distribution are satisfied. More general methods such as Bayesian estimation make it possible to estimate the parameters without requiring that the assumptions of the multilevel models be satisfied. In addition, the Bayesian estimation is robust to a small sample size, a situation that is more likely to occur in higher level observations, and in general, it is able to deal with technical problems such as multicollinearity of the data.

In this chapter, we adapted the bottom-up strategy to specify a multilevel model in the frequentist approach to the Bayesian approach. Our proposal was to use the Bayesian LOO-CV between the different steps for the comparison of models. Deviance information criterion (DIC) could also be used instead of Bayesian LOO-CV.

Two factors had a significant association with probing depth. Bleeding (site-level covariate) and dental calculus (patient-level covariate). At the tooth level, a factor associated with the probing depth was not found.

The methodology set out in this chapter can be applied to other areas of the health sciences with data with a hierarchical structure and numerical response variable.

Acknowledgements

Tino-Salgado is indebted to CONACYT for fellowship that enabled him to pursue graduate studies for the degree of Maestría en Matemáticas Aplicadas. The authors thank the sixth semester periodontics students of the 2013–2018 batch for their assistance and logistical support during the patient recruitment stage.

Conflict of interest

The authors declare no conflict of interest.

Abbreviations

DIC	Deviance information criterion
HMC	Hamiltonian Monte Carlo
ESS	Effective sample size
GEE	Generalized estimating eqs.
GR	Gelman and Rubin diagnostic
ICC	Intraclass correlation coefficient
LOO-CV	Leave-one-out cross-validation
lppd	Log pointwise predictive density
MCMC	Markov chain Monte Carlo
MGLM	Multilevel generalized linear models
NUTS	No-U-turn sampling
PSRF	Potential scale reduction factor

Author details

Edilberta Tino-Salgado[1†], Flaviano Godínez-Jaimes[1†], Cruz Vargas-De-León[1,2*], Norma Samanta Romero-Castro[3], Salvador Reyes-Fernández[3] and Victor Othon Serna-Radilla[3]

1 Facultad de Matemáticas, Maestría en Matemáticas Aplicadas, Universidad Autónoma de Guerrero, Chilpancingo de los Bravo, Mexico

2 División de Investigación, Hospital Juárez de México, Ciudad de México, Mexico

3 Facultad de Odontología, Especialidad en Implantología y Rehabilitación Bucal, Universidad Autónoma de Guerrero, Acapulco, Mexico

*Address all correspondence to: leoncruz82@yahoo.com.mx

† These authors contributed equally.

References

[1] Kim JS, Kim D-K, Hong SJ. Assessment of errors and misused statistics in dental research. International Dental Journal. 2011;**61**(3): 163-167

[2] Wang J, Xie H, Fisher JF. Multilevel Models, Applications Using SAS. Berlin, Germany: de Gruyter; 2011. DOI: 10.1515/9783110267709

[3] Joop J Hox, Mirjam Moerbeek y Rens Van de Schoot. Multilevel Analysis: Techniques and Applications. New York, United States: Routledge; 2017

[4] Gilks WR, Richardson S, Spiegelhalter D. Markov Chain Monte Carlo in Practice. Florida, United States: CRC Press; 1995

[5] Matthew D Hoffman, Andrew Gelman y col. The No-U-turn sampler: Adaptively setting path lengths in Hamiltonian Monte Carlo. The Journal of Machine Learning Research 2014;**15**(1): 1593–1623

[6] Bürkner P-C. brms: An R package for Bayesian multilevel models using stan. Journal of Statistical Software. 2017;**80**(1):1-28. DOI: 10.18637/jss.v080.i01

[7] Roy V. Convergence diagnostics for markov chain Monte Carlo. Annual Review of Statistics and Its Application. 2020;7:387-412

[8] Plummer M, Best N, Cowles K, Vines K. CODA: Convergence diagnosis and output analysis for MCMC. R News. 2006;**6**(1):7-11

[9] Gelman A, Carlin JB, Stern HS, Dunson DB, Vehtari A, Rubin DB. Bayesian Data Analysis. Florida, United States: CRC Press; 2013

[10] Romero-Castro NS, Castro-Alarcon N, Reyes-Fernández S, Flores-Alfaro E, Parra-Rojas I. Periodontal disease distribution, risk factors, and importance of primary healthcare in the clinical parameters improvement. International Journal of Odonto Stomatology. 2020;**14**(2):183-190. DOI: 10.4067/S0718-381X2020000200183

[11] Bürkner P-C. Advanced Bayesian multilevel modeling with the R package brms. The R Journal. 2018;**10**(1):395-411. DOI: 10.32614/RJ-2018-017

[12] Carpenter B, Gelman A, Hoffman MD, Lee D, Goodrich B, Betancourt M, et al. Stan: A probabilistic programming language. Journal of Statistical Software. 2017;**76**(1):1-32. DOI: 10.18637/jss.v076.i01

[13] Holmes Finch W, Bolin JE, Kelley K. Multilevel Modeling Using R. CRC Press; 2019

Section 2

Spatial Statistics

Chapter 6

Spatial Modeling in Epidemiology

María Guzmán Martínez, Eduardo Pérez-Castro, Ramón Reyes-Carreto and Rocio Acosta-Pech

Abstract

The objective of this chapter is to present the methodology of some of the models used in the area of epidemiology, which are used to study, understand, model and predict diseases (infectious and non-infectious) occurring in a given region. These models, which belong to the area of geostatistics, are usually composed of a fixed part and a random part. The fixed part includes the explanatory variables of the model and the random part includes, in addition to the error term, a random term that generally has a multivariate Gaussian distribution. Based on the random effect, the spatial correlation (or covariance) structure of the data will be explained. In this way, the spatial variability of the data in the region of interest is accounted for, thus avoiding that this information is added to the model error term. The chapter begins by introducing Gaussian processes, and then looks at their inclusion in generalized spatial linear models, spatial survival analysis and finally in the generalized extreme value distribution for spatial data. The review also mentions some of the main packages that exist in the R statistical software and that help with the implementation of the mentioned spatial models.

Keywords: Geostatistic, gaussian process, spatial GLM, spatial survival analysis, spatial extremes

1. Introduction

The term spatial statistics is used to describe a wide range of statistical models and methods for the analysis of geo-referenced data [1]. Its rapid use has been increasing in various fields of science, such as biology, image processing, environmental and earth sciences, ecology, epidemiology, agronomy, forestry, among others [2]. In epidemiology, spatial statistics are used to study the occurrence of health-disease events or deaths in a region of interest. It is now known that several public health problems tend to exhibit spatial dependence (spatial autocorrelation, spatial variability), and that sometimes these problems are related to climatic factors that are generally of a spatially continuous nature or with factors specific to the study region. The use of classical statistical techniques to model spatial data generally leads to an overestimation of model parameters [1]; and although they may eventually help, these models, lacking adequate structure, will not be able to model the spatial variability of the data; valuable information that will be sent to model error and cannot be used to explain the nature of the phenomenon under study.

Recent studies have shown that spatial models can help identify spatial patterns in infectious and non-infectious diseases. These models also help determine the factors that favor them, such as sociodemographic, environmental, etc.; as well as generate maps to visualize the distribution of morbidity or mortality of infectious and non-infectious diseases, and identify critical points in the spatial distribution [3, 4].

Generalized linear spatial models (GLSM), which are a particular class of multilevel or hierarchical models, have been used for the study of certain diseases (infectious and non-infectious). The estimation of GLSM parameters can be done under the frequentist or Bayesian approach [1], some examples are given below. A spatial Poisson regression model, where parameter estimation was performed under the frequentist approach, was used to study esophageal cancer incidence rates [5] and the sociodemographic risk factors for diabetes [6]. Under the Bayesian approach, these models have been used to study the relationship between Visceral Leishmaniasis incidence rates and climatological variables [7], as well as to identify risk factors associated with nontuberculous mycobacterial infections [8]. Spatial Binomial regression models, under the Bayesian approach, have been used to describe patterns of occurrence of dengue and chikungunya [9], and filariasis [10]. Under the classical approach, spatial binomial regression models have been used to investigate environmental and sociodemographic factors associated with leptoserosis disease [11]; are also used to study risk factors associated with HIV infection among drug users [12].

On the other hand, survival analysis under the spatial approach has also received great attention in recent years, because geographic location can play a relevant role in predicting disease survival [13]. Fragility models (spatial survival models) can be an option to analyze the heterogeneity of the data when it cannot be explained by the covariates in a classical survival model. In spatial survival models, in addition to covariates, a random effect known as *frailty* is added, which modifies the hazard function of an individual, or of spatially correlated individuals [14]. Generally, the random factor, which is assigned a multivariate normal distribution, plays an important role in modeling survival times; since in this term the differences that exist in the socioeconomic level, access to medical care, population density, weather conditions, among others, can be taken into account. It is worth mentioning that spatial survival models have been applied in studies such as: recovery time in patients with COVID-19 [15], hospitalization time in dengue patients [16], HIV/AIDS survival [17] and breast cancer [18] to name a few. In all these works, the estimation of the model parameters was under the Bayesian approach.

Extreme events in public health (for example, the saturation of hospitals) are generally analyzed through measures of central tendency or time series, however, these approaches are not the most appropriate to understand extreme events (unusual events); that when they occur they strongly impact the health care network, thus often collapsing the system [19]. The extreme value theory (EVT) aims to study the probability of occurrence of extreme events (values) of a phenomenon of interest over time, generally these values only occur when they exceed a threshold. Although the applications of EVT in public health are scarce, if they exist at all; an application was presented when predicting extreme events of annual seasonal influenza mortality and the number of emergency department visits in a network of hospitals [20], another application was presented when modeling elevated cholesterol levels using the spikes-over-threshold model [21]. In both cases, the parameters were estimated under the frequentist approach. Given the advantages they have with the application of a spatial model, it would be convenient to study the extreme events of the health sector in space, for which there is already a methodology known as spatial modeling of extreme values [22].

The objective of this work is to provide a general review of the theoretical framework of spatial statistical models developed in the area of geostatistics, which have been used in the area of epidemiology to analyze, model and predict the phenomena of interest. Some of the packages that exist in the statistical software R [23] to carry out said spatial analyzes are also mentioned.

2. Gaussian processes

A stochastic process $W(t), t \in T$ is a collection of random variables. That is, for each $t \in T$, $W(t)$ is a random variable [24]; if the stochastic process is indexed by a coordinate space $s \in A \subset \mathbb{R}^d$, then the stochastic process is called a random field [25]. A realization of the random field, $W(s), s \in A$, is given by $(W(s_1) = y(s_1), \dots, W(s_n) = y(s_n))$. Generally from the sample $y(s_1), \dots, y(s_n)$ one tries to know the characteristics of the process W in s_i, $i = 1, \dots, n$; and with this information to make inference of the process $W(s)$ on all $A \subset \mathbb{R}^d$, a convex set where s varies continuously. To the geo-referenced data $y(s_1), \dots, y(s_n)$ is often referred to as geocoded, geostatistical data or point-referenced data. The study of this type of data is known as geostatistics, which is a part of spatial statistics that studies phenomena with continuous variation in space, a convex region denoted A [26].

A process W is second order stationary if it has finite variance, constant mean and its covariance function depends only on distance. Having second-order stationarity in a stochastic process implies having intrinsic stationarity, i.e., second-order stationarity is stronger than intrinsic stationarity. On the other hand, weak stationarity and second-order stationarity are equivalent in the space [27]. The following defines what is known as a Gaussian process (field).

Definition 1. A stochastic process $\{W(s) : s \in A \subset \mathbb{R}^2\}$, where s varies continuously on a fixed subset A content in $\mathbb{R}^2$, is a Gaussian process if for any collection of locations $s_1, \dots, s_n$ with $s_i \in A$, the joint distribution of $(W(s_1), \dots, W(s_n))$ is multivariate Gaussian [1].

What is known as a stationary Gaussian process is defined below.

Definition 2. A Gaussian process $\{W(s) : s \in A \subset \mathbb{R}^2\}$, is stationary if $\forall s \in A$:

$$E(W(s)) = 0, \tag{1}$$

$$Var(W(s)) = \sigma^2, \tag{2}$$

and its correlation function depends only on the distance, i.e.

$$Corr(W(s), W(s')) = \rho(h), \tag{3}$$

where $h = \|s - s'\|$ is the Euclidean distance that exists between s and s'.

That is, the mean and variance of $W(s)$ are constant and its correlation function only depends on the distance, so that

$$W \sim \mathcal{N}(0, \sigma^2 \rho(h)) \tag{4}$$

Given $\mathbf{W} = (W_1, \dots, W_n)$, where $W_i = W(s_i)$, the distribution of $\mathbf{W}$ is normal multivariate $(\mathcal{NM})$, i.e.

Family	Correlation function
Exponential	$\rho(h,\phi) = \exp\left(-\frac{h}{\phi}\right)$
Gaussian	$\rho(h,\phi) = \exp\left(-\frac{h^2}{\phi^2}\right)$
Spherical	$\rho(h,\phi) = 1 - 1.5\left(\frac{h}{\phi}\right) + 0.5\left(\frac{h}{\phi}\right)^3$
Circular	$\rho(h,\phi) = 1 - \frac{2}{\pi}\left(a\sqrt{1-a^2} + \sin^{-1}\sqrt{a}\right)$
Cubic	$\rho(h,\phi) = 1 - \left[7\left(\frac{h}{\phi}\right)^2 - \frac{35}{4}\left(\frac{h}{\phi}\right)^3 + \frac{7}{2}\left(\frac{h}{\phi}\right)^5 - \frac{3}{4}\left(\frac{h}{\phi}\right)^7\right]$
Wave	$\rho(h,\phi) = \frac{\phi}{h}\sin\left(\frac{h}{\phi}\right)$
Matérn	$\rho(h,\phi,\kappa) = \frac{1}{2^{\kappa-1}\Gamma(\kappa)}\left(\frac{h}{\phi}\right)^{\kappa} K_\kappa\left(\frac{h}{\phi}\right)$
Powered exponential	$\rho(h,\phi,\kappa) = \exp\left[-\left(\frac{h}{\phi}\right)^{\kappa}\right]$
Cauchy	$\rho(h,\phi,\kappa) = \left[1 + \left(\frac{h}{\phi}\right)^2\right]^{-\kappa}$
Stable	$\rho(h,\phi,\kappa) = \exp\left(-\frac{h}{\phi}\right)$
Bessel	$\rho(h,\phi,\kappa) = \left(\frac{2\phi}{h}\right)^{\kappa}\Gamma(\kappa+1)J_\kappa\left(\frac{h}{\phi}\right)$

Table 1.
Models for the spatial correlation structure of a spatial process.

$$\mathbf{W} \sim \mathcal{NM}(\mathbf{0}, \sigma^2\mathbf{R}), \tag{5}$$

where the (i,j) element of $\mathbf{R}$ is given by $(\mathbf{R})_{ij} = Corr(W(s_i), W(s_j)) = \rho(h_{ij}), h_{ij} = \|s_i - s_j\|$ is the Euclidean distance between s_i and s_j. Note that the covariance of the Gaussian process is given by $Cov(\mathbf{W}) = \sigma^2\mathbf{R}$.

In this way, the correlation structure of a stationary Gaussian process can be studied through the $\rho(h)$ function. Several parametric expressions for this function are shown in the **Table 1**. In these correlation functions, $\phi > 0$ is a range parameter controlling the spatial decay over distance; $h = \|s - s'\|$ is the Euclidean distance between s and s' and $h \geq 0$; $\Gamma(\cdot)$ denotes the gamma function. $\kappa > 0$, in theory of spatial extremes $J_\kappa(\cdot)$ and $K_\kappa(\cdot)$ are the Bessel and modified Bessel function of the third kind of order κ [28], while in the spatial survival analysis and generalized linear models $K_\kappa(\cdot)$ is the modified Bessel function of the second kind of order κ [29]; κ is a shape parameter that determines the analytic smoothness of the underlying process W [1]. In the powered exponential correlation function $0 < \kappa \leq 2$ and in the Bessel correlation function $\kappa \geq 0$.

3. Gaussian spatial model

Generally from process $\{W(s) : s \in A \subset \mathbb{R}^2\}$, there is a noisy version, i.e., a set of observation $y(s_1), \ldots, y(s_n)$ of the random variables $Y(s_1), \ldots, Y(s_n)$, $s_i \in A$. In this way $Y(s)$ is a measurement process of $W(s)$, $s \in A$ [1, 26].

The Gaussian geostatistical model, in the absence of independent variables, is given by

$$Y(s) = \mu + W(s) + Z(s), \quad s \in A, \tag{6}$$

where μ is a constant mean effect, $W(s)$ is a stationary Gaussian process (1) and $Z(s)$ is the error term in the model with $Z(s) \sim \mathcal{N}(0, \tau^2)$; τ^2 is the nugget effect variance. $Z(s)$ is known as measurement error, micro-scale variation or a non-identifiable combination of the two [22, 26].

Thus for a realization of a stationary Gaussian spatial process, $\mathbf{Y}(s) = (Y(s_1), \dots, Y(s_n))$, $s_i \in A$ and $i = 1, \dots, n$ with

$$Y(s_i) = \mu + W(s_i) + Z(s_i), \tag{7}$$

where

- $W(s_i) \sim \mathcal{N}(0, \sigma^2)$.
- $Z(s_i)$ are mutually independent and identically distributed, $Z(s_i) \sim \mathcal{N}(0, \tau^2), \; i = 1, \dots, n$.
- $Z(s_i)$ are independent of the process $W(\cdot)$ [26].
- Conditional on $W(\cdot)$, random variables $Y(s_i)$, $i = 1, \dots, n$, are mutually independent with normal distribution,

$$Y(s_i)|W(\cdot) \sim \mathcal{N}\left(\mu + W(s_i), \tau^2\right). \tag{8}$$

The joint distribution of $\mathbf{Y}(s)$ is normal multivariate given by

$$\mathbf{Y}(s) \sim \mathcal{NM}\left(\mu\mathbf{1}, \sigma^2\mathbf{R}(\phi) + \tau^2\mathbf{I}\right), \tag{9}$$

where

- μ is the mean of the Gaussian process $W(\cdot)$ and $\mathbf{1}$ is a vector of dimension $n \times 1$.
- σ^2 is the variance of the process $W(\cdot)$.
- $\mathbf{R}(\phi)$ is a matrix of correlations of dimension $n \times n$, whose elements given by

$$(\mathbf{R}(\phi))_{ij} = \rho_Y\left(h_{ij}, \phi\right), \tag{10}$$

where $h_{ij} = \left\|s_i - s_j\right\|$ is the euclidean distance that exists between s_i and s_j that are in A, and ϕ is a spatial scale parameter.

- τ^2 is the variance of Z and $\mathbf{I}$ is the identity matrix of dimension $n \times n$.
- Note that the covariance of the $\mathbf{Y}(s)$ is given by $Cov(\mathbf{Y}(s)) = \sigma^2\mathbf{R}(\phi) + \tau^2\mathbf{I}$.

When $\mathbf{Y}(s)$ can be explained by a set of covariates that also depend on the location, $\mathbf{X}(s) = \left(X_1(s), \dots, X_p(s)\right)$, then the model is given by

$$\mathbf{Y}(s) = \mathbf{X}(\mathbf{s})\beta + \mathbf{W}(s) + \mathbf{Z}(s), \quad s \in A, \tag{11}$$

with

$$\mathbf{Y}(s) \sim \mathcal{NM}\left(\mathbf{X}(\mathbf{s})\beta, \ \sigma^2\mathbf{R}(\phi) + \tau^2\mathbf{I}\right), \tag{12}$$

where $\beta = \left(\beta_0, \ldots, \beta_p\right)$ is a vector of unknown regression parameters; in this case also $Cov(\mathbf{Y}(s)) = \sigma^2\mathbf{R}(\phi) + \tau^2\mathbf{I}$. The unknown parameters in this model are β, σ^2, τ^2 and ϕ. The parameters of the Models (4) y (5) can be estimated under the classical approach (maximum likelihood or maximum restricted likelihood) and under the Bayesian statistical approach [1, 30]. Among the most important points in geostatistics is the modeling of the covariance structure of the spatial process and the identification of the interpolation method that will be used to perform the prediction of the process in the non sampled points in A. Regarding the last point, [31] made a compilation of the most used criteria for assessing the performance of the spatial interpolation method.

The *geoR* package contains the *likfit* function that allows to estimate, under Maximum likelihood (ML) or restricted maximum likelihood (REML), the parameters of a Gaussian process [32]. The function *likfit* estimates the coefficients of the models (4) y (5).

The function *krige.cov* of the same package helps to perform the spatial prediction of a Gaussian process using simple kriging (SK), ordinary kriging (OK), external trend kriging (KTE) and universal kriging (UK) [33]. The package *glmmfields* allows to fit Gaussian models [34] under the Bayesian approach.

On the other hand, with the function *glmmfields* of the package *glmmfields*, the coefficients of the models (4) and (5) can be estimated under the Bayesian approach. The function *glmmfields* reports the posterior median of the parameters with their respective 95% credible intervals; this function, also reports the values of the Gelman and Rubin statistic [35], where values less than 1.20 would indicate convergence of the chain.

4. Generalized linear spatial models

Generalized linear models (GLM) [36, 37] are very useful when the response variable does not follow a normal distribution. The assumptions of GLMs are

1.1. $Y_i, i = 1, \ldots, n$ are mutually independent with expectations μ_i.

2. The μ_i are specified by $g(\mu_i) = \eta_i$, where $g(\cdot)$ is a known link function.

3. The linear predictor is given by $\eta_i = x_i'\beta$, where x_i is a vector of explanatory variables associated with the response Y_i, and β is a vector of unknown parameters.

The Y_i follow a common distributional family, indexed by their expectations μ_i, and possibly by additional parameters common to all n responses.

An important extension of this basic class of models is the generalized linear mixed model (GLMM) [38], in which $Y_1, \ldots, Y_n$ are mutually independent conditional on the realized values of a set latent random variables (random effects) $U_1, \ldots, U_n$ and the conditional expectations are given by $g(\mu_i) = U_i + x_i'\beta$. A generalized linear spatial model is a GLMM in which the $U_1, \dots, U_n$ are derived from spatial process. Diggle and Ribeiro in 2007 [1], refers to these models as generalized linear geostatistical model (GLGM). In accordance with Diggle et al. [39], the assumptions of the generalized linear spatial models are as follows

1. W is a stationary Gaussian process, $W \sim \mathcal{N}(0, \sigma^2\rho(h))$, (Eq. (1)).

2. Conditionally an W, the random variables Y_i, $i = 1, \dots, n$ are mutually independent, with distributions $f_i(y|W(s_i)) = f(y; M_i)$, specified by the values of the conditional expectations $M_i = E[Y_i|W(s_i)]$.

3. $g(M_i) = \mathbf{x}_i'\beta + W(s_i)$ for some known link function g and explanatory variable $\mathbf{x}_i = \mathbf{x}(s_i)$.

Then $M_i = g^{-1}(\mathbf{x}_i'\beta + W(s_i))$, where the linear predictor would be given by $\eta_i = \mathbf{x}_i'\beta + W(s_i)$.

Taking Diggle and Tawn as a precedent (1998) [39]; Jing and De Oliveira in 2015 [40] state the GLSM as follows

$$Y_i|W_i \sim p(\cdot|\mu_i). \tag{13}$$

where

$$\mathbf{W} \sim \mathcal{NM}(\mathbf{X}\beta, \sigma^2\mathbf{R}) \tag{14}$$

R is of the same form as the Gaussian process (2)

- $Y(s_i) : i = 1, \dots, n$ are conditionally independent given **W** with pdfs or pmfs $p(\cdot|\mu_i)$.
- $E(Y_i|W_i) = \mu_i$ and $g(\cdot)$ is a known one-to-one link function.
- $\mathbf{X} = (\mathbf{1}, \mathbf{x}_1, \dots, \mathbf{x}_p)$ is a known $n \times (p + 1)$ design matrix assumed of full-rank, with **1** a vector of $n \times 1$ of ones and $\mathbf{x}_j = (x_j(s_1), \dots, x_j(s_n))'$, where $x_j(s_i)$ is the value of the j-th covariate of the i-th sampling location, and $\beta = (\beta_0, \beta_1, \dots, \beta_p)$ is the vector of unknown regression parameters.

Since g is the link function then $g(\mu_i) = \eta_i$ and $\mu_i = g^{-1}(\eta_i)$, $i = 1, \dots, n$, where the linear predictor is given by $\eta_i = W_i$, then $\mu_i = g^{-1}(W_i)$. The unknown parameters in GLSM are β, σ^2 and ϕ.

The two most widely used GLSM for spatial count data are the Poisson and Binomial spatial models [39, 41].

The *geoCount* [40] package implements the GLSM; the function *runMCMC* is used to generate posterior samples of the Gaussian process and the GLSM parameters, with which the parameter estimates and their credibility intervals can be obtained.

In the package *geoRglm* [42, 43], the functions *glsm.krige*, *pois.krige* and *binom.krige* implement the GLSMs, in this case, parameter estimation is performed under the frequentist approach. While the functions *krige.bayes*, *pois.krige.bayes* and *binom.krige.*

bayes, which also implement the GLSMs, estimate the parameters under the Bayesian approach. These functions report estimates of β, σ^2 and ϕ.

The *glmmfields* package implements the Gamma, Poisson, Negative Binomial, Binomial and Lognormal models using the function *glmmfields* [34], parameter estimation is performed under the Bayesian approach. The function *glmmfields* reports the parameter estimates using the posterior median with their respective 95% percentile credible intervals; it also reports the Gelman and Rubin diagnostic values.

5. Spatial survival models

Generally, survival analysis models are specified through their hazard function, $h(t)$, whose intuitive interpretation is that $h(t)\delta t$ is the conditional probability that a patient will die in the interval $(t, t + \delta t)$, given tat they have survived until time t. The most widely used approach to modeling $h(t)$, at least in medical applications, is to use a semi-parametric formulation [44]. In this approach, the hazard for the i-th patient is modeled as

$$h(t_i) = h_0(t_i)\exp\left(x_i'\beta\right), \tag{15}$$

where x_i is a vector of explanatory variables for patient i and $h_0(t)$ is an unspecified baseline hazard function. This is known as a proportional hazards (PH) model, because for any two patients i and j, $h(t_i)/h(t_j)$ does not change over time [1].

Another key idea in survival analysis is frailty, this corresponds to the random effects term used; time-to-event data will be group into strata, such as clinical sites, geographic regions, etc. This gives rise to mixed models, which include a random effect (the frailty) that correspond to a stratum's overall health status [30]. To illustrate, let t_{ij} be the time to death or censoring for subject j in stratum i, $j = 1, \dots, n_i$, $i = 1, \dots, m$. Let $\mathbf{x}_{ij}$ be a vector of individual specific covariates, then

$$h(t_{ij}, x_{ij}) = h_0(t_{ij})\exp\left(\mathbf{x}_{ij}'\beta + W_i\right), \tag{16}$$

where W_i es the stratum-specific frailty term, designed to capture differences among strata; strata are typically denoted by s_i, $i = 1, \dots, m$, so s_i denotes the location of the i-th patient and $W_i = W(s_i)$. It can be assumed that the W_i are independent identical distribution (iid), i.e.

$$W_i \sim \mathcal{N}(0, \sigma^2). \tag{17}$$

But it can also be assumed that W_i arises from a Gaussian process, i.e. if $\mathbf{W} = (W_1, \dots, W_m)$, then

$$\mathbf{W} \sim \mathcal{NM}(\mathbf{0}, \sigma^2\mathbf{R}(\phi)). \tag{18}$$

This way, suppose subjects are observed at m distinct spatial locations $s_1, \dots, s_m \in A$. Let t_{ij} be a random event time associated with the j-th subject in s_i, assume the survival time t_{ij} lies in the interval (a_{ij}, b_{ij}), $i = 1, \dots, m$, $j = 1, \dots, n_i$; and $\mathbf{x}_{ij}$ be a related p-dimensional vector of covariates, then are defined proportional hazard (PH) frailty models, accelerated failure time (AFT) frailty models and proportional odds (PO) frailty models.

PH frailty models are the extensions of the population hazards model which is best known as the Cox model [44] a widely pursued model in survival analysis. PH frailty models extends the Cox model such that the hazard of an individual depends in addition on an unobserved random variable W, then introducing an additive frailty term W_i for each individual in the exponent of the hazard function as follows

$$h\left(t_{ij}, \mathbf{x}_{ij}\right) = h_0\left(t_{ij}\right)e^{\mathbf{x}'_{ij}\beta + W_i}. \tag{19}$$

The corresponding survival function and the density are given by

$$\begin{aligned} S\left(t_{ij}, \mathbf{x}_{ij}\right) &= S_0\left(t_{ij}\right)^{e^{\mathbf{x}'_{ij}\beta + W_i}}, \\ f\left(t_{ij}, \mathbf{x}_{ij}\right) &= e^{\mathbf{x}'_{ij}\beta + W_i} S_0\left(t_{ij}\right)^{e^{\mathbf{x}'_{ij}\beta + W_i} - 1} f_0\left(t_{ij}\right), \end{aligned} \tag{20}$$

where $S_0(\cdot)$, $f_0(\cdot)$ and $h_0(\cdot)$ are the baseline survival function, baseline density and baseline hazard function assumed to be unique for all individual in the study population respectively.

Accelerated failure time frailty model extends the AFT model such that the hazard of an individual depends in addition on an unobserved random variable W [45–47]. Introducing an additive frailty term W_i for each individual in the exponent of the hazard function it becomes:

$$h\left(t_{ij}, \mathbf{x}_{ij}\right) = h_0\left(e^{\mathbf{x}'_{ij}\beta + W_i} t_{ij}\right)e^{\mathbf{x}'_{ij}\beta + W_i}. \tag{21}$$

The survival function and density are given by

$$\begin{aligned} S\left(t_{ij}, \mathbf{x}_{ij}\right) &= S_0\left(e^{\mathbf{x}'_{ij}\beta + W_i} t_{ij}\right), \\ f\left(t_{ij}, \mathbf{x}_{ij}\right) &= e^{\mathbf{x}'_{ij}\beta + W_i} f_0\left(e^{\mathbf{x}'_{ij}\beta + W_i} t_{ij}\right), \end{aligned} \tag{22}$$

where $S_0(\cdot)$, $f_0(\cdot)$ and $h_0(\cdot)$ are the baseline survival function, baseline density and baseline hazard function assumed to be unique for all individual in the study population respectively.

Finally, proportional odds frailty model is given by

$$h\left(t_{ij}, \mathbf{x}_{ij}\right) = h_0 \frac{1}{1 + \left[e^{-\mathbf{x}'_{ij}\beta - W_i} - 1\right] S_0\left(t_{ij}\right)}. \tag{23}$$

The survival function and density are given by

$$\begin{aligned} S\left(t_{ij}, \mathbf{x}_{ij}\right) &= \frac{S_0\left(t_{ij}\right)e^{-\mathbf{x}'_{ij}\beta - W_i}}{1 + \left(e^{-\mathbf{x}'_{ij}\beta - W_i} - 1\right) S_0\left(t_{ij}\right)}, \\ f\left(t_{ij}, \mathbf{x}_{ij}\right) &= \frac{f_0\left(t_{ij}\right)e^{-\mathbf{x}'_{ij}\beta - W_i}}{\left[1 + \left(e^{-\mathbf{x}'_{ij}\beta - W_i} - 1\right) S_0\left(t_{ij}\right)\right]^2}, \end{aligned} \tag{24}$$

where $S_0(\cdot)$, $f_0(\cdot)$ and $h_0(\cdot)$ are the baseline survival function, baseline density and baseline hazard function assumed to be unique for all individual in the study population respectively.

In the frailty models, it is possible to deal with left, right and interval censoring of the data. Among the packages that exist in the R statistical software to perform spatial survival analysis is the *spBayesSurv* package [48]; the function *survregbayes* estimates the parameters of the PH, AFT and PO spatial models under the classical and Bayesian approach; also reports the posterior mean and median of the regression coefficients and of the parameters of the covariance function of the Gaussian process, σ^2 and ϕ, with their 95% credible intervals. The *spBayesSurv* package uses the powered exponential function (Table 0) to model the spatial correlation of the data.

Also in R, there is the *spatsurv* package [49], which implements the function *survspat* that fits parametric PH spatial survival models. This function reports the estimates and posterior median of the parameters β, σ^2 and ϕ with the respective credibility intervals.

6. Spatial generalized extreme value model

According to Coles (2001) [50], given $Y_1, \ldots, Y_n$ a sequence of independent random variables with a common distribution function F with $M_n = \max\{Y_1, \ldots, Y_n\}$, if there a sequences of constants $a_n > 0$ and b_n such that

$$P((M_n - b_n)/a_n \leq z) \rightarrow G(z), \tag{25}$$

when $n \rightarrow \infty$, for a non-degenerative distribution function G, then G is a member of the generalized extreme value (GEV) distribution family

$$G(y;\eta,\tau,\xi) = \exp\left\{-\left[1+\xi\left(\frac{y-\eta}{\tau}\right)\right]^{\frac{-1}{\xi}}\right\}, \tag{26}$$

defined on $\{z : 1+\xi(z-\eta)/\tau > 0\}$, where $-\infty < \eta < \infty$, $\tau > 0$ and $-\infty < \xi < \infty$.

Davison et al. in 2012 [51], describe spatial GVE as follows. For each s in $\mathbb{R}^2$, suppose that $Y(s)$ is GEV distributed whose parameters $\mu(s)$, $\sigma(s)$ and $\xi(s)$ vary smoothly for s in $\mathbb{R}^2$ according to a stochastic process $W(s)$. We assume that the processes for each GEV parameters are mutually independent Gaussian processes [52]. Then

$$\begin{aligned} \eta(s) &= f_\eta(s;\beta_\eta) + W_\eta(s;\sigma_\eta,\phi_\eta,\kappa_\eta), \\ \tau(s) &= f_\tau(s;\beta_\tau) + W_\tau(s;\sigma_\tau,\phi_\tau,\kappa_\tau), \\ \xi(s) &= f_\xi(s;\beta_\xi) + W_\xi(s;\sigma_\xi,\phi_\xi;\kappa_\xi), \end{aligned} \tag{27}$$

where f_η, f_τ and f_{xi} are deterministic functions depending on a regression parameters β_η, β_τ and β_ξ respectively. While W_η, W_τ and W_ξ are a zero mean stationary Gaussian process with correlation function $\rho(h,\phi_\eta,\kappa_\eta)$, $\rho(h,\phi_\tau,\kappa_\tau)$ and $\rho(h,\phi_\xi,\kappa_\xi)$ respectively, i.e.

$$\begin{aligned} W_\eta &\sim \mathcal{N}\left(0,\sigma_\eta^2\rho(h,\phi_\eta,\kappa_\eta)\right), \\ W_\tau &\sim \mathcal{N}(0,\sigma_\tau^2\rho(h,\phi_\tau,\kappa_\tau)), \\ W_\xi &\sim \mathcal{N}\left(0,\sigma_\xi^2\rho(h,\phi_\xi,\kappa_\xi)\right). \end{aligned} \tag{28}$$

Then conditional on the values of the tree Gaussian process at the sites $(s_1, \dots, s_k)$, the maxima are assumed to follow GEV distributions

$$Y_{s_i}|\eta(s_j), \tau(s_j), \xi(s_j) \sim GEV(\eta(s_j), \tau(s_j), \xi(s_j)) \quad (29)$$

z independently for each location $s_1, \dots, s_k, j = 1, \dots, k$ and $i = 1, \dots, n$.

Davison *et al.* in 2012 [51], proposed the construction of Bayesian hierarchical models for spatial extremes.

The *SpatialExtremes* package [53] allows modeling spatial extremes, through max-stable processes with the function *fitmaxstab*, which reports the values of the parameter estimates with their respective standard errors.

To implement hierarchical Bayesian models, the function *latent* is used, this reports the posterior median of the scale, shape and location parameters with their respective credible intervals.

Another package in the literature to model spatial extremes is *glmmfields* [34], with the function *glmmfields*, parameter estimation is performed under the Bayesian approach. The function *glmmfields* also allows modeling spatial extreme events incorporating temporally, that is, time, these models are known as spatio-temporal models.

7. Conclusions

The main characteristic of spatial data is that observations close in space tend to be correlated, and in spatial modeling this correlation is used to understand the behavior of the phenomenon under study in a region of interest.

Omitting the spatial dependence of the data can generate a bias of the information and, consequently, lead to an incorrect inference. Therefore, adequately describing the spatial pattern of an event can provide sufficient elements to elaborate possible hypotheses of its cause. As we have seen, the spatial variability of georeferenced data can be studied with the spatial models developed in geostatistics. The usefulness of these models has been demonstrated in several applications related to the identification of social structures, disease patterns, occupational patterns, as well as in the identification of populations (or subgroups) that are at greater or lesser risk of an event. As we have seen, in statistics, all correctly processed information helps in correct decision making. In this sense, this paper aims to introduce the reader to the use of spatial models in geostatistics.

If the response or variable of interest is the cases (counts) of sick people in a given region, or the new cases of a disease in a given period of time (incidence), then Poisson GLSMs can be useful to know the spread of the disease in the population of interest, predict new cases, and identify the variables that influence the occurrence of the disease. On the other hand, when the response variable is a binary or ratio variable, such as mortality rates or infection rates, then binomial GLSMs can be helpful. These models have been used to study the prevalence of dengue and to identify the variables associated with the event.

Conflict of interest

The authors declare no conflict of interest.

Abbreviations

AFT	Accelerated failure time
EVT	Extreme value theory.
GEV	generalized extreme value.
GLSM	Generalized Linear Spatial Models.
GLM	Generalized linear models.
GLMM	generalized linear mixed model
GLGM	generalized linear geostatistical model
iid	Independent identical distribution
$\mathcal{NM}$	Normal multivariate.
PH	Proportional hazards.
PO	Proportional odds.

Author details

María Guzmán Martínez[1*†], Eduardo Pérez-Castro[1†], Ramón Reyes-Carreto[1] and Rocio Acosta-Pech[2]

1 Universidad Autónoma de Guerrero, Chilpancingo de los Bravo, México

2 Colegio de Postgraduados, Tabasco, México

*Address all correspondence to: manguzgm@gmail.com

† These authors contributed equally.

References

[1] Diggle PJ, Ribeiro PJ. Model-Based Geostatistics. New York: Springer; 2007. p. 228

[2] Gaetan C, Guyon X. Spatial Statistics and Modeling. New York, NY: Springer Science+Business Media, LLC; 2010

[3] Rezaeian M, Dunn G, St. Leger S, Appleby L. Geographical epidemiology, spatial analysis and geographical information systems: A multidisciplinary glossary. Journal of Epidemiology and Community Health. 2007;**61**(2):98-102. DOI: 10.1136/jech.2005.043117

[4] Chowell G, Rothenberg R. Spatial infectious disease epidemiology: On the cusp. BMC Medicine. 2018;**16**(1):1-5. DOI: 10.1186/s12916-018-1184-6

[5] Mohebbi M, Wolfe R, Jolley D. A poisson regression approach for modelling spatial autocorrelation between geographically referenced observations. BMC Medical Research Methodology. 2011;**11**(1):1-11. DOI: 10.1186/1471-2288-11-133

[6] Kauhl B, Schweikart J, Krafft T, Keste A, Moskwyn M. Do the risk factors for type 2 diabetes mellitus vary by location? A spatial analysis of health insurance claims in Northeastern Germany using kernel density estimation and geographically weighted regression. International Journal of Health Geographics. 2016;**15**(1):1-12. DOI: 10.1186/s12942-016-0068-2

[7] Ben-Ahmed K, Aoun K, Jeddi F, Ghrab J, El-Aroui MA, Bouratbine A. Visceral leishmaniasis in Tunisia: Spatial distribution and association with climatic factors. The American Journal of Tropical Medicine and Hygiene. 2009;**81**(1):40

[8] Lipner EM, Knox D, French J, Rudman J, Strong M, Crooks JL. A geospatial epidemiologic analysis of nontuberculous mycobacterial infection: An ecological study in Colorado. Annals of the American Thoracic Society. 2017;**14**(10):1523-1532

[9] Hira FS, Asad A, Farrah Z, Basit RS, Mehreen F, Muhammad K. Patterns of occurrence of dengue and chikungunya, and spatial distribution of mosquito vector Aedes albopictus in Swabi district, Pakistan. Trop Med Int Heal. 2018;**23**(9):1002-1013. DOI: 10.1111/tmi.13125

[10] Slater H, Michael E. Mapping, Bayesian geostatistical analysis and spatial prediction of lymphatic filariasis prevalence in Africa. PLoS One. 2013;**8**(8):28-32. DOI: 10.1371/journal.pone.0071574

[11] Mayfield HJ, Lowry JH, Watson CH, Kama M, Nilles EJ, Lau CL. Use of geographically weighted logistic regression to quantify spatial variation in the environmental and sociodemographic drivers of leptospirosis in Fiji: A modelling study. Lancet Planet Heal. 2018;**2**(5):223-232. DOI: 10.1016/S2542-5196(18)30066-4

[12] Zhou YB, Wang QX, Liang S, Gong YH, Yang MX, Chen Y, et al. Geographical variations in risk factors associated with HIV infection among drug users in a prefecture in Southwest China. Infectious Diseases of Poverty. 2015;**4**(1):1-10. DOI: 10.1186/s40249-015-0073-x

[13] Zhou H, Hanson T, Zhang J. SpBayesSurv: Fitting bayesian spatial survival models using R. Journal of Statistical Software. 2020;**92**(9):1-33. DOI:10.18637/jss.v092.i09

[14] Banerjee S, Wall MM, Carlin BP. Frailty modeling for spatially correlated survival data, with application to infant mortality in Minnesota. Biostatistics. 2003;**4**(1):123-142. DOI: 10.1093/biostatistics/4.1.123

[15] Mahanta KK, Hazarika J, Barman MP, Rahman T. An application of spatial frailty models to recovery times of COVID-19 patients in India under Bayesian approach. Journal of Scientific Research. 2021;**65**(03):150-155. DOI: 10.37398/JSR.2021.650318

[16] Aswi A, Cramb S, Duncan E, Hu W, White G, Mengersen K. Bayesian spatial survival models for hospitalisation of dengue: A case study of Wahidin hospital in Makassar, Indonesia. International Journal of Environmental Research and Public Health. 2020;**17**(3):1-12. DOI: 10.3390/ijerph17030878

[17] Martins R, Silva GL, Andreozzi V. Bayesian joint modeling of longitudinal and spatial survival AIDS data. Statistics in Medicine. 2016;**35**(19):3368-3384. DOI: 10.1002/sim.6937

[18] Zhou H, Hanson T, Jara A, Zhang J. Modeling county level breast cancer survival data using a covariate-adjusted frailty proportional hazards model. The Annals of Applied Statistics. 2015;**9**(1):43-68. DOI: 10.1214/14-AOAS793

[19] Chiu Y, Chebana F, Abdous B, Bélanger D, Gosselin P. Mortality and morbidity peaks modeling: An extreme value theory approach. Statistical Methods in Medical Research. 2018;**27**(5):1498-1512. DOI: 10.1177/0962280216662494

[20] Thomas M, Lemaitre M, Wilson ML, Viboud C, Yordanov Y, Wackernagel H, et al. Applications of extreme value theory in public health. PLoS One. 2016;**11**(7):3-9. DOI: 10.1371/journal.pone.0159312

[21] De Zea BP, Mendes Z. Extreme value theory in medical sciences: Modeling total high cholesterol levels. J Stat Theory Pract. 2012;**6**(3):468-491. DOI: 10.1080/15598608.2012.695673

[22] Gelfand AE, Schliep EM. Spatial statistics and gaussian processes: A beautiful marriage. Spatial Statistics. 2016;**18**:86-104. DOI: 10.1016/j.spasta.2016.03.006

[23] R Core Team. R: A Language and Environment for Statistical Computing. Vienna, Austria: R Foundation for Statistical Computing; 2021. URL https://www.R-project.org/

[24] Ross SM et al. Stochastic Processes. Vol. 2. New York: Wiley; 1996

[25] Grigoriu M. Stochastic processes. In: Calculus S, editor. Birkhäuser. Boston: MA; 2002. pp. 103-204

[26] Diggle PJ, Ribeiro PJ, Christensen OF. An introduction to model-based geostatistics. In: Møller J, editor. Spatial Statistics and Computational Methods. New York: Springer Verlag; 2003. pp. 43-86

[27] Cressie N, Wikle CK. Statistics for Spatio-Temporal Data. John Wiley & Sons; 2015

[28] Ribatet M. A user's Guide to the SpatialExtremes Package. Lausanne, Switzerland: EPFL; 2009

[29] Chilès JP, Delfiner P. Geostatistics: Modeling Spatial Uncertainty. New York: Wiley Series In Probability and Statistics; Vol. 497; 2009

[30] Banerjee S, Carlin BP, Gelfand AE. Hierarchical Modeling and Analysis for Spatial Data. 2nd ed. United States of America: Chapman and Hall/CRC; 2004. p. 472

[31] Li J, Heap A. A review of comparative studies of spatial interpolation methods in environmental sciences: Performance and impact factors. Ecol Inform. 2011;**6**(3–4): 228-241. DOI: 10.1016/j.ecoinf.2010.12.003

[32] Ribeiro PJ, Diggle PJ. geoR: A package for geostatistical analysis. R-NEWS. 2001;**1**:15-18

[33] Goovaerts P. Geostatistics for Natural Resources Evaluation. New York: Oxford University Press; 1997

[34] Anderson SC, Ward EJ. Black swans in space: Modeling spatiotemporal processes with extremes. Ecology. 2019; **100**(1):1-23. DOI: 10.1002/ecy.2403

[35] Gelman A, Rubin DB. Inference from iterative simulation using multiple sequences. Statistical Science. 1992;7(4): 457-511. DOI: 10.1214/ss/1177011136

[36] Nelder J, Wedderburn R. Generalized linear models. Journal of the Royal Statistical Society Series A (General). 1972;**135**(3):370-384. DOI: 10.2307/2344614

[37] McCullagh P, Nelder JA. Generalized Linear Models. 2nd ed. London: Chapman and Hall; 1989

[38] Breslow NE, Clayton DG. Approximate inference in generalized linear mixed models. Journal of the American Statistical Association. 1993; **88**(421):9-25

[39] Diggle PJ, Tawn JA, Moyeed RA. Model-based geostatistics. Journal of the Royal Statistical Society: Series C (Applied Statistics). 1998;**47**(3):299-350

[40] Jing L, De Oliveira V. Geocount: An R package for the analysis of geostatistical count data. Journal of Statistical Software. 2015;**63**:1-33. DOI: 10.18637/jss.v063.i11

[41] Christensen OF, Waagepetersen R. Bayesian prediction of spatial count data using generalized linear mixed models. Biometrics. 2002;**58**(2):280-286. DOI: 10.1111/j.0006-341x.2002.00280.x

[42] Christensen OF, Ribeiro PJ Jr. geoRglm-a package for generalised linear spatial models. R News. 2002;**2**(2):26-28

[43] Ribeiro PJ Jr, Christensen OF, Diggle PJ. geoR and geoRglm: Software for model-based geostatistics. Hornik K, Leisch F, Zeileis A, editors. Vienna: 3rd International Workshop on Distributed Statistical Computing (DSC 2003): 20-22 March 2003; p. 2

[44] Cox DR. Regression models and life-tables. J R Stat Soc [B]. 1972;**34**(2): 187-202. DOI: 10.1111/j.2517-6161.1972.tb00899.x

[45] Buckley J, James I. Linear regression with censored data. Biometrika. 1979; **66**(3):429-436. DOI: 10.2307/2335161

[46] Wei L. The accelerated failure time model: A useful alternative to the cox regression model in survival analysis. Statistics in Medicine. 1992;**11**(14–15): 1871-1879. DOI: 10.1002/sim.4780111409

[47] Zhang J, Lawson AB. Bayesian parametric accelerated failure time spatial model and its application to prostate cancer. Journal of Applied Statistics. 2011;**38**(3):591-603. DOI: 10.1080/02664760903521476

[48] Zhou H, Hanson T, Zhang J. spBayesSurv: Fitting Bayesian Spatial Survival Models Using R. 2017. arXiv preprint arXiv:1705.04584

[49] Taylor BM, Rowlingson BS. Spatsurv: An R package for bayesian

inference with spatial survival models. Journal of Statistical Software. 2017;**77**(4):1-32. DOI:10.18637/jss.v077.i04

[50] Coles S, Bawa J, Trenner L, Dorazio P. An Introduction to Statistical Modeling of Extreme Values. Vol. 208. London: Springer; 2001. p. 208

[51] Davison AC, Padoan SA, Ribatet M. Statistical modeling of spatial extremes. Statistical Science. 2012;**27**(2):161-186. DOI: 10.1214/11-STS376

[52] Casson E, Coles S. Spatial regression models for extremes. Extremes. 1999; **1**(4):449-468. DOI: 10.1023/A:1009931222386

[53] Ribatet M. SpatialExtremes: An R Package for Modelling Spatial Extremes. R Package Version 2.1-0. 2020. Available from: https://cran.r-project.org/web/packages/SpatialExtremes/

Chapter 7

Spatial Statistics in Vector-Borne Diseases

Manuel Solís-Navarro, Susana Guadalupe Guzmán-Aquino, María Guzmán-Martínez and Jazmín García-Machorro

Abstract

Vector-borne diseases are those caused by the bite of an infected arthropod, such as the *Aedes aegypti* mosquito, which can infect humans with dengue or Zika. Spatial statistics is an interesting tool that is currently implemented to predict and analyze the behavior of biological systems or natural phenomena. In this chapter, fundamental characteristics of spatial statistics are presented and its application in epidemiology is exemplified by presenting a study on the prediction of the dispersion of dengue disease in Chiapas, Mexico. A total of 573 confirmed dengue cases (CDCs) were studied over the period of January–August 2019. As part of the spatial modeling, the existence of spatial correlation in CDCs was verified with the Moran index (MI) and subsequently the spatial correlation structure was identified with the mean squarer normalized error (MSNE) criterion. A Generalized Linear Spatial Model (GLSM) was used to model the CDCs. CDCs were found to be spatially correlated, and this can be explained by a Matérn covariance function. Finally, the explanatory variables were maximum environmental temperature, altitude, average monthly rainfall, and patient age. The prediction model shows the importance of considering these variables for the prevention of future CDCs in vulnerable areas of Chiapas.

Keywords: vector-borne diseases, Gaussian process, generalized spatial linear models, georeferenced data, spatial correlation

1. Introduction

Vector-borne diseases are infections caused by viruses, bacteria, or parasites that are transmitted to humans by the bite of infected arthropod species, these can be diseases transmitted by mosquitoes (dengue fever, West Nile fever, chikungunya, malaria, Zika, etc.), by sandflies (leishmaniasis), by ticks (encephalitis, Lyme Borreliosis, Crimean-Congo hemorrhagic fever, Human Granulocytic Anaplasmosis) by triatomines (Chagas disease), among others. These diseases account for more than 17% of all infectious diseases and cause more than 700, 000 deaths per year [1, 2].

Vectors are living organisms that can transmit infectious pathogens between humans or from animals to humans. Many of these vectors are insects that ingest disease-causing microorganisms during a blood meal from an infected host and then transmit it to a new host after the pathogen has replicated. Another characteristic of arthropod vectors is that they are cold-blooded (ectothermic) and therefore very sensitive to climatic factors, although the climate is only one of many factors that influence vector distribution, as there are also geographic and sociodemographic factors [1].

In order to interpret the behavior of vector-borne diseases in the most accurate and simplified way possible, statistical models are used. A statistical model is a simplified representation of a phenomenon of interest [3, 4]. With their help, it is possible to model, predict and make inferences about natural phenomenons, biological systems, epidemiological studies, and others [5]. One of the most widely used statistical models is linear regression models, which predict a continuous target based on linear relationships between the target and one or more predictors. But there is another type of model that extends the general linear model, so that the dependent variable is linearly related to the factors and covariates by means of a certain link function, which is known as a generalized linear model [6].

Generalized Linear Models (GLMs) provide a collection of linear regression models including the exponential family, such as the Binomial and Poisson, which are distributions for counting data. The GLMs were introduced by Nelder in 1972 [7], in 1989 they were studied in greater depth by McCullagh [8] and over time more authors were integrated [9–13].

There are three components in GLMs: A response variable distribution, a linear predictor, and a link function. A response variable $\mathbf{Y}$ is assumed $(Y_1, Y_2, \dots, Y_n)$, where $Y_1, Y_2, \dots, Y_n$ are independent of each other; its expected value is related to a linear predictor $E[Y] = g^{-1}(\mathbf{d}'\boldsymbol{\beta})$, where $\boldsymbol{\beta} \in \Re^p$ is a vector of regression parameters, $\mathbf{d}$ are known explanatory variables and g is a known function called a link function, which allows to define the relationship between the systematic and random components [14].

GLMs can help in numerous areas such as epidemiology, mining engineering, Earth and environmental sciences, ecology, biology, geography, economics, agronomy, forestry, image processing, and more [15, 16]. For epidemiology in particular, as it is about understanding diseases that affect a population, the most usual thing is to find a binary variable that represents the presence or absence of a disease or to count the events of a disease for certain areas.

Such is the case of a study conducted by Hashizume et al. [17] in Bangladesh, 2012. They used a Generalized Linear Poisson Regression Model to examine weekly dengue hospitalizations in relation to river levels, during the years 2005 to 2009, and the climatic variables daily precipitation and average temperature. The models were adjusted according to seasonal variation and temperature. They found evidence of a 6.9% increase in dengue with high river levels, but a 29.6% increase in disease when rivers were very low.

An important extension of the GLMs is the Generalized Linear Mixed Models (GLMMs) [18]. GLMMs provide a range of analyses for those data that are correlated in space and belong to the exponential family (Gamma, Poisson, Binomial, among others) [19]. Generalized Linear Spatial Models (GLSMs) are basically GLMMs, since latent variables are derived from a spatial process. In recent years, there has been a growing interest in the analysis of spatial data in epidemiology, in order to predict the incidence of vector-borne diseases.

Using techniques available to epidemiologists and other health professionals, the potential of remote sensing, Geographic Information Systems (GIS), and spatial analysis of epidemiological data has been demonstrated by some authors such as those mentioned below; however, there are still few studies that adequately prove the potential of these tools, since they are still being exploited in the fight against diseases [20].

For instance, a Colombian paper published in 2012, Sanchez et al. [21] estimated Generalized Linear Spatial Regression Models with a Poisson response to explain the behavior of malaria and dengue in different years. Health determinants were identified in the occurrence of these diseases and risk maps were obtained. Finally, it demonstrated the need to link spatial effects in the models and the explanatory variables considered, to explain the number of reported cases of the disease in the years analyzed.

Another example is the work of Estallo et al. [22] in 2021, which evaluated the species responsible for the transmission of *Leishmaniasis* (phlebotom-*Phlebotominae*) during the period 2012 − 2014 in northern Argentina. Through Generalized Linear Mixed Models, the implications of vectors in disease transmission were evaluated, using meteorological and teledetection environmental factors. It was observed that the species *Lutzomyia* longipalpis was the most abundant in urban areas. The findings allowed detecting of high-risk areas and the developing of predictive models to optimize resources and prevent *leishmaniasis* transmission in the area.

As can be seen, spatial analysis is a powerful tool for the analysis of georeferenced data, as it can give health research a broader perspective of the occurrence of health events and diseases. Spatial statistical models are useful because they estimate the spatial variance inherent in the data, and can also be used to perform statistical inference throughout the study area. Spatial prediction can be made based entirely on a stochastic model or in combination with a deterministic trend [20, 23].

The aim of this chapter is to show an example of the application of spatial statistics, implementing a Generalized Linear Spatial Model for the prediction of dengue disease in the state of Chiapas. For this, there are considered patient age and the next information of each municipality: garbage disposal service, maximum environmental temperature, average monthly rainfall, and altitude as covariates. For the study of the disease in the 118 municipalities of Chiapas, the cases observed in 36 municipalities in the state of Chiapas and the information in the aforementioned explanatory variables were considered.

2. Spatial statistical models

Space models have a simple structure, flexible enough to handle a variety of problems. The data may be continuous or discrete, present spatial aggregations, or be point observations in space. As for the spatial locations can be regular or irregular. A spatial model is usually used to predict sites where the study phenom was not observed.

Let $x \in A \subset \mathbb{R}^d$ and $S(x)$ the data observed at the x location, this results in a stochastic process

$$S(x) : x \in A \tag{1}$$

Structure 1, allows to differentiate and talk about problems with continuous spatial indexes, lattice, and point patterns giving rise to three types of data: geospatial, lattice data, and point patterns. In geospatial data, A is a fixed set in $\mathbb{R}^d$ containing a d-dimensional rectangular with positive volume; $S(x)$ is a random vector in the location $x \in A$. These data arise in areas such as atmospheric sciences, mining, and public health. In point patterns A is a point process in $\mathbb{R}^d$ or a subset of $\mathbb{R}^d$; $S(x)$ is a random vector in the location $x \in A$. In its most general form, it results in a spatial point process marked when $S(x) = 1$, for all $x \in A$. Point patterns arise when the variable to be analyzed is a location of "events".

Finally, the entangled data or also known as area data, A is a regular or irregular fixed set (with additional information from the surrounding neighborhood) of $\mathbb{R}^d$; $S(x)$ is a random vector in location $x \in A$. When locations are in regular meshes it is the closest analogy to time series observed at equally spaced time points. In the entangled data, based on the general spatial process 1, it is assumed that A is an accounting collection of space sites, in which the data are observed. The most common entangled data models are the Conditional Autoregressive Model (CAR) and the Simultaneous Autoregressive Model (SAR). CAR models form the basis of Markovian Gaussian random fields and Integrated Nested Laplace Approximation (INLA) methods. SAR models are popular in geographic information systems. Other models are the spatial autoregressive moving average (ARMA) [24, 25].

2.1 Gaussian spatial processes

Knowing the type of variables with which they are working and taking into account their spatial dependence, helps to determine the regression technique that best fits the characteristics of the data [21]. For the study of spatial data Gaussian processes can be used, which are stochastic processes, a collection of variables. This allows any subset of finite random variables to have a multivariate Gaussian distribution. Gaussian processes can thus be thought of as distributions of random vectors or random functions [26]. Gaussian processes began to be studied in the 1940s, but until the 1970s they were used in geostatistics and meteorology; In the 1990s Cressie [24] began to implement them in spatial statistics. In fact, the term "model-based geostatistics" was first used to describe an approach to geostatistical problems based on formal statistical models and inference procedures [27].

Gaussian stochastic processes are widely used as models for geostatic data. If a transformation of the original response variable is used, the scope of the Gaussian models can be amplified, and so with this extra flexibility the model provides a good empirical fit to the data.

A Gaussian process, $\{S(x) : x \in \mathbb{R}^2\}$, is a stochastic process with the property that for any collection of locations $x_1, \dots, x_n$, $x_i \in \mathbb{R}^2$, the joint distribution of $\mathbf{S} = \{S(x_1), \dots, S(x_n)\}$ is multivariate Gaussian.

Any such process is fully specified by the average function $\mu(x) = E[S(x)]$ and the covariance function $Cov\{S(x), S(x')\}$. As given $x_1, \dots, x_n$ an arbitrary set of locations with $\boldsymbol{\mu} = (\mu(x_1), \dots, \mu(x_n))$ and $\mathbf{G}$ an $n \times n$ matrix with elements $G_{ij} = Cov(S(x_i), S(x_j))$; then $\mathbf{S}$ has a multivariate normal distribution (MN).

$$\mathbf{S} \sim MN(\boldsymbol{\mu}, \mathbf{G}) \tag{2}$$

A spatial Gaussian process is stationary if $\mu(x)$ is constant, $\mu(x) = \mu$, for all x and $Cov(S(x), S(x')) = Cov(u)$; where $u = \|x - x'\|$ is the Euclidean distance. A stationary process is isotropic if the covariance between the values of $S(x)$ at any two locations depends only on the distance between them. The term stationary is often used as the equivalence of stationary and isotropic. A process for which $S(x) - \mu(x)$ is stationary is called covariance stationary. Processes of this type are widely used in practice as models for geostatistical data [28].

Among the parametric functions for the covariance function [29] are the following:

Exponential:

$$Cov(u) = \sigma^2 \left[\exp\left(\frac{-u}{\phi}\right) \right] \tag{3}$$

Gaussian:

$$Cov(u) = \sigma^2 \left[\exp\left(-\frac{u}{\phi}\right)^2 \right] \tag{4}$$

Matérn:

$$Cov(u) = \sigma^2 \left[\frac{2}{2^{\kappa-1}\Gamma(\kappa)} \left(\frac{u}{\phi}\right)^{\kappa} K_{\kappa}\left(\frac{u}{\phi}\right) \right] \tag{5}$$

In these covariance functions (Eqs. (3)–(5)) $u > 0$, $\phi > 0$, y $\kappa > 0$; function K_κ denotes the modified Bessel function of order κ and $\Gamma(\cdot)$ denotes the gamma function.

2.2 Criteria for evaluating the covariance structure of the Gaussian process

There are several criteria in the literature to validate the covariance structure of a Gaussian process Eq. (2). Among the most used are: Mean Error (ME), Mean Square Error (MSE), Mean Absolute Error (MAE), Root Mean Square Error (RMSE) and Mean Square Normalized Error (MSNE) (**Table 1**). ME and MSE should tend to zero when the covariance structure of the Gaussian process was correctly estimated. The MAE and RMSE criteria are considered as the most efficient criteria to validate the covariance structure of the Gaussian process. The RMSE is expected to be small like MAE, while the MSNE is expected to be close to 1 [29, 30].

Measurement	Definition
Mean error	ME=$\frac{1}{n}\sum_{i=1}^{n}\left(Y(s_i) - \hat{Y}(s_i)\right)$
Mean square error	MSE=$\frac{1}{n}\sum_{i=1}^{n}\left(Y(s_i) - \hat{Y}(s_i)\right)^2$
Mean absolute error	MAE=$\frac{1}{n}\sum_{i=1}^{n}\left(\lvert Y(s_i) - \hat{Y}(s_i)\rvert\right)$
Root mean square error	RMSE=$\left[\frac{1}{n}\sum_{i=1}^{n}\left(Y(s_i) - \hat{Y}(s_i)\right)^2\right]^{\frac{1}{2}}$
Mean square normalized error	MSNE =$\frac{1}{n}\sum_{i=1}^{n}\frac{\left(Y(s_i)-\hat{Y}(s_i)\right)^2}{\hat{\sigma}^2_{ok}(s_i)}$

$\hat{\sigma}^2_{ok}$ is a variance estimated by the ordinary kriging interpolation method [29].

Table 1.
Criteria for evaluating the covariance structure of the Gaussian process.

2.3 Generalized linear spatial models

Spatial Generalized Linear Models were introduced by Diggle et al. in 1998 [31]; if the variable response Y has Poisson distribution, then

$$Y_i|S(\cdot) \sim Poisson(\mu_i) \tag{6}$$

Where

$$\mathbf{S} \sim MN(\mathbf{D}\beta, \mathbf{G})$$

It is assumed that $\{Y_i : i = 1, \dots, n\}$ conditioned in $\mathbf{S}$ are independent, $E[Y_i|S(\cdot)] = \mu_i$, gs a known link function such that $g(\mu_i) = \eta_i$ then $\mu_i = g^{-1}(\eta_i)$, $i = 1, \dots, n$. $\mathbf{D} = (\mathbf{1}, \mathbf{d}_1, \dots, \mathbf{d}_p)$ is a design matrix of $n \times (p+1)$ of full range, $\mathbf{1}$ a vector $n \times 1$ of ones and $\mathbf{d}_j = (d_j(x_1), \dots, d_j(x_n))'$, where $d_j(x_i)$ is the value of the covariate j-th of the i-th location; $\beta = (\beta_0, \beta_1, \dots, \beta_p)$ the regression parameters.

2.4 Moran's index for spatial autocorrelation

To prove the existence of spatial dependence on a variable Y, the Moran index [32, 33], given by

$$IM = \frac{n\sum_i^n \sum_i^n w_{ij}\left(Y_i - \overline{Y}\right)\left(Y_i - \overline{Y}\right)}{\sum_{i \neq j}^n w_{ij} \sum_i^n \left(Y_i - \overline{Y}\right)^2} \tag{7}$$

Where $\mathbf{W}$ is the weights matrix that defines the relationships between the regions of the study. In this case $w_{ij} = 1$ denotes areas with a common border and $w_{ij} = 0$ in another case. Y_i and Y_j would be the values observed in regions i and j respectively, while $\overline{Y}$ is the average incidence of the districts studied, n is the total number of localities.

2.5 Statistical software packages R for spatial data

Several packages are available in statistical software R [34] to perform spatial modeling.

The *geoR* package is used for performing geostatistical data analysis and spatial prediction, which expands the set of methods and tools presently available for spatial data analysis in R. The package executes methods for Gaussian and Gaussian models transformed, incorporates functions and methods for reading and preparing the data, exploratory analysis, inference on model parameters and spatial interpolation, and it also contains functions for parameter estimation under Bayesian methods [35].

The *geoRglm* package is used to implement Generalized Linear Spatial Model. The subsequent and predictive inference is based on Markov Chains Monte Carlo (MCMC) methods. This package, which is an extension of the *geoR* package, help with GLSM conditional simulation and prediction, and with Bayesian inference for the models Poisson (*pois.krige*) and Binomial (*binom.krige*) [35, 36]. A Langevin-Hastings algorithm is used to obtain MCMC simulations. In the *pois.krige* and *binom.krige* functions, the user can provide a value for the variation of the proposal *S.scale*, a value initial, *S.start*, the thinning, *thin*, the length of the burn, *burn.in*, and the number of iterations, *n.iter* [35].

2.5.1 Inference for the generalized linear spatial model

The geostatistical model assumes the response variable to be Gaussian, which may be an unrealistic assumption for some data sets. The GLSM provides a framework for analyzing Binomial and Poisson distributed data. The likelihood for such a model, in general, cannot be represented in closed form, since it is a high-dimensional integral

$$L(\boldsymbol{\beta}, \sigma^2, \phi) = \int \prod_{i=1}^{n} f\left(y_i; g^{-1}(s_i)\right) p\left(s; \boldsymbol{\beta}, \sigma^2, \phi\right) ds \tag{8}$$

where $f(y;\mu)$ denotes the density of the distribution with mean μ, $p(s;\boldsymbol{\beta},\sigma^2,\phi)$ is the multivariate Gaussian density for the vector **s** of random effects at the data locations and $g(\cdot)$ is the link function. In practice, the high dimensionality of this integral precludes direct computation, so the inference is based on MCMC.

3. Description of data

This section shows the application of a spatial model taking into account the social, climatic, and geographical characteristics of the municipalities of the state of Chiapas in relation to dengue virus infections registered from January to August of the year 2019.

3.1 Study area

Dengue disease is endemic to the state of Chiapas with scattered case reports, this is due to the different geographic characteristics of the state, such as the altitude of its municipalities and its border condition with the country of Guatemala. It is known that at different altitudes, in the regions, the climatic conditions tend to vary and this can favor the reproduction of the vector. The state of Chiapas is divided into 118 municipalities, each with different sociodemographic and climatic conditions. The population density, according to the INEGI, is around 5, 544 million inhabitants; being the state capital, Tuxtla Gutiérrez, the municipality with the highest population density; for the year 2019, 604, 147 inhabitants were registered [37].

3.2 Data collection

The data, which were collected at the municipal level, being 36 the municipalities that registered positive cases of dengue and were considered for the analysis, were obtained from different sources that are mentioned below.

3.2.1 Dengue cases

The database with dengue cases registered in the state of Chiapas, during the period January–August 2019, was obtained from the Secretary of Health of the state of

Chiapas, in collaboration with the area of vector-borne diseases. This database is updated week by week, fulfilling 52 Epidemiological Weeks (EW) reports per year.

3.2.2 Climatic data

The climatic data were obtained from the World Meteorological Organization (WMO) [38], for each municipality of residence where the dengue cases were registered, working with the daily reports of average environmental temperature, maximum and minimum environmental temperature and average monthly rainfall. The climatic data were taken into account for the analysis, 6 days before the onset of symptoms for each case, this was done considering the intrinsic incubation period in order to obtain an approximate date of infection and capture the daily climatic data for each municipality [39]. With respect to the rainfall variable, it was decided to work with the monthly average, since there were days in which there were no records.

3.2.3 Non-climatic data

Other factors related to infection were also considered in the analysis. Data on the population density and altitude of each municipality of residence per observed case were obtained from the INEGI, the other variables such as garbage disposal, contact with the mosquito, drinking water service, patient age, and sex were obtained from the original database of registered dengue cases provided by the secretary of health [37].

3.3 Georeferencing

For the georeferencing of dengue cases registered in the period January–August 2019, the postal code and the world geographic coordinate system, WGS84, were used. With the *pois.krige* function from the *geoRglm* package, in R software version 4.0.3 [34] and the projection of the cases was carried out on a map of Chiapas.

4. Results

The database that is made up of 573 dengue cases, reported in the state of Chiapas, Mexico, during the period January–August of the year 2019; being the state capital, (Tuxtla Gutiérrez) the municipality with the highest number of CDCs, with 49.04%, the rest of the cases were scattered in other 35 municipalities of the State. The average age of the cases was 14 years, with the female sex being the most affected with 53%, in the same way, 15% indicated not having the drinking water service.

4.1 Spacial location

The spatial distribution of the 573 dengue cases is heterogeneous in 36 municipalities in the state of Chiapas (blue points in **Figure 1**).

4.2 Moran's index

The Moran's Index obtained, with the number of CDCs in the 36 municipalities of Chiapas, was 0.115, which indicates that there is a spatial relationship in the number

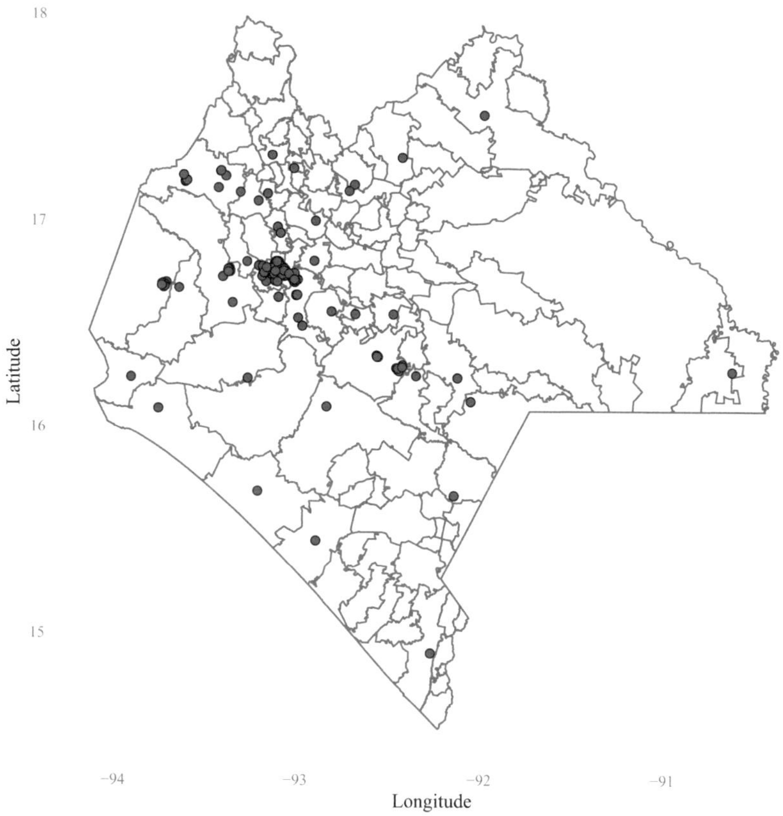

Figure 1.
Georeferencing of cases 573 DCs registered in Chiapas.

of cases observed in the municipalities ($p - value = 0.001$). Therefore, it is convenient to study the CDCs with a spatial model, since it is a counting variable, a Generalized Linear Spatial Model was used.

4.3 Evaluation of the covariance structure of georeferenced data

After selecting the spatial model and the variables, we proceeded to estimate the covariance structure of the Gaussian process. For this, the Exponential, Gaussian, and Matérn covariance functions were tested, taking CDCs as the response variable, and measures of central tendency of the explanatory variables maximum environmental temperature, altitude, patient age, and average monthly rainfall were taken. Of the three functions, the Matérn covariance function generated the best value for $ME = -1.185$ and $MSNE = 0.885$, that is, ME tends to 0 and $MSNE$ tends to 1, therefore a covariance function Matérn can be assumed for the fitted spatial model.

4.4 Parameter estimation

For the simulation and conditional prediction of the process Eq. (6) MCMC was used, since this provides a solution to the impediment of direct calculation of the

Parameter	Estimation coeff.	95% Confidence intervals
Intercept (β_0)	1.88952	$(1.88178, 1.96555)$
Maximum temp. (β_1)	0.00740	$(0.00523, 0.00763)$
Altitude (β_2)	0.00028	$(0.00026, 0.00028)$
Rainfall (β_3)	−0.02549	$(-0.02607, -0.02423)$
Age (β_4)	−0.05356	$(-0.05444, -0.05275)$

Table 2.
Estimation of parameters and their confidence intervals of the selected model.

predictive distribution due to the high dimensionality of the integral Eq. (8) [36]. For this, 505000 simulations were performed, with a burn-in period of 5000 data and a thinning of chains of 100 data. Ordinary kriging was used for data interpolation. The initial values for the GLSM parameters were $\sigma^2 = 3$, $\phi = 0.5$ and $\beta = (0.1, 0.1, 0.1, 0.1)$. The estimation of β was carried out under the classical approach. Confidence intervals at 95% were obtained using 1000 Monte Carlo simulated samples [40].

For modeling the number of registered dengue cases in the 36 municipalities of Chiapas, Y_i, $i = 1, \dots, 36$. As for the 13 covariates considered, only the variables maximum environmental temperature, altitude above sea level in the municipality, average monthly rainfall, and patient age showed a relationship with the number of confirmed dengue cases. It was verified that the problem of multicollinearity did not exist in those included in the model: altitude and maximum environmental temperature ($r = -0.2231, p - value = 0.191$), average monthly rainfall and maximum temperature ($r = 0.243, p - value = 0.1534$), average monthly rainfall and altitude ($r = 0.1724, p - value = 0.3147$).

In **Table 2**, it is observed that the variables that have an effect on the cases of dengue observed are maximum environmental temperature, altitude of the municipalities, average monthly rainfall, and patient age. High temperatures and altitudes favor the presence of the disease, while young people will be preferred factors by the vector, as well as low rainfall because in seasons where there is no continuous flow of water in the rivers, stagnation causes an increase in the proliferation of *Aedes* mosquitoes.

4.5 Prediction of the model to the Chiapas map

The projection of the model was carried out on a map of the state of Chiapas which was made based on the municipalities where the cases were registered, as can be seen in **Figure 2**, the prediction is divided by zones in shades of green to yellow with a contour delimited by contour lines that show the area in which the model predicts the number of cases for that area. As we can see, most of the predicted cases occur within the metropolitan area where the state capital Tuxtla Gutiérrez and the municipalities of Chiapa de Corzo, Berriozábal and Suchiapa are located, this corresponds to the observed data, since most of the cases occurred in the same area. On the other hand, it is observed that the prediction power is diminished in areas where no dengue cases were registered.

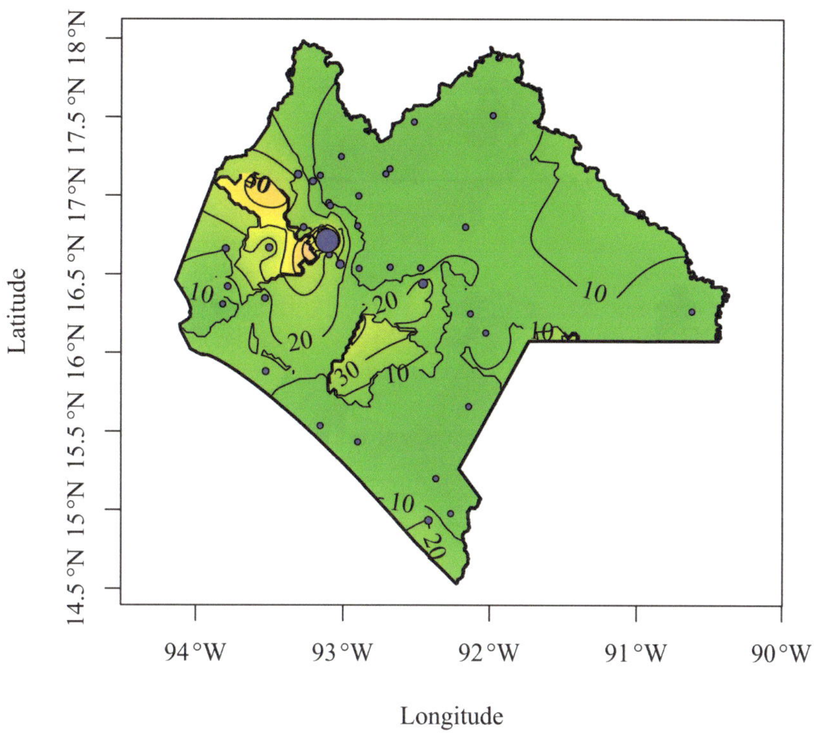

Figure 2.
Prediction of confirmed dengue cases.

5. Discussion

The purpose of this chapter is to present and expand the use of spatial statistics to contribute to public health and the epidemiology of vector-borne diseases, and for this reason, the example of the use of a GLSM was proposed to model the distribution of dengue in Chiapas, since this is one of the endemic diseases that cause numerous infections per year. Climatological, geographic, and sociodemographic variables were used for the modeling, where it was found that the maximum environmental temperature, altitude, patient age, and average monthly rainfall are the variables that best predict the spread of dengue.

Maximum environmental temperature is shown to have a significant effect on dengue cases, as it is an environmental risk factor for dengue transmission, higher temperatures increase viral replication in the vector in a shorter time and thus increase the potential for transmission of dengue viruses. This is described by a study on the extrinsic incubation period. Liu et al. [41] found that the virus remained in the midgut of the vector at 18°C, but could spread and invade the salivary glands at temperatures between 23°C and 32°C, thus demonstrating that higher temperatures create a shorter extrinsic incubation period and greater transmission potential.

The altitude above sea level of each municipality was also an important variable in the study, which is consistent with the findings of the systematic review by Aswi [42], where this variable was used in different statistical models in order to describe the behavior of the disease, since the spread of the Aedes aegypti mosquitoes is limited by climatic conditions and this will be governed by the location of the geographical area and its altitude. The study of Reinhold et al. [43] alludes that Aedes Aegytpi cannot regulate its body temperature because it is an endothermic arthropod, and that is why its temperature is defined by the climatic conditions of its environment. Thus, geographic location and altitude are important variables for dengue disease.

On the other hand, we have average monthly rainfall, where we see a negative association, since the less rainfall, the more cases of dengue. This coincides with the results of the work of Hashizume et al. [17], where they indicate that dengue cases increase by 29.6% in the months when the rivers have low flow, and this is understandable, since, in those seasons of the year when rainfall is scarce, the rivers do not have a continuous flow of water, which produces stagnation and these, in turn, become ideal breeding grounds for mosquitoes, causing an increase in the proliferation of Aedes.

Finally, we have the variable patient age, as can be seen in the results, the correlation was negative too, due to the young population being preferred by the vector, since there is a greater number of cases at an average age of 14 years. As demonstrated by Phanitchat et al. [44] in their work, where it was reported that the age range of dengue cases was between 5 and 14 years in northeastern Thailand.

6. Conclusions

Vector-borne diseases (VBD) are an important public health issue worldwide. The distribution of these diseases as well as their transmission and seasonality are known to be largely determined by environmental, geographic, and socio-demographic factors. GLSMs allow robust analysis of the complex and diverse factors that influence the occurrence of VBD, incorporating spatial dimensions. They can also be a valuable tool for targeting interventions in surveillance and control programs for VBD at the global or regional level. These analytical approaches have recently been used in the field of public health, but in Mexico there are still very few studies that contribute to this knowledge. For this reason, this chapter presents an example of the application of GLSM with a study of dengue, one of the most common VBD in Mexico, finding that the maximum temperature, altitude, and average monthly rainfall of each municipality, as well as patient age, are the factors that best predicted the presence of dengue cases in the state of Chiapas in the period from January to August 2019.

Conflict of interest

The authors declare no conflict of interest.

Abbreviations

ARMA	Autoregressive Moving Average
CAR	Conditional Autoregressive Model
CDCs	Confirmed Dengue Cases
DENV	Dengue Virus
EW	Epidemiological Week
GLM	Generalized Linear Model

GLMM	Generalized Linear Mixed Model
GLSM	Generalized Linear Spatial Model
INEGI	National Institute of Statistic and Geography
INLA	Integrated Nested Laplace Approximation
MAE	Mean Absolute Error
MCMC	Markov Chain Monte Carlo
ME	Mean Error
MI	Moran's Index
MSE	Mean Square Error
MSNE	Mean Square Normalized Error
RMSE	Root Mean Square Error
SAR	Simultaneous Autoregressive Model
VBD	Vector-Borne Diseases
WMO	World Meteorological Organization
ZCL	Zoonotic Cutaneous *Leishmaniasis*

Author details

Manuel Solís-Navarro[1†], Susana Guadalupe Guzmán-Aquino[1†], María Guzmán-Martínez[2*] and Jazmín García-Machorro[1]

1 Instituto Politécnico Nacional, Escuela Superior de Medicina, Ciudad de México, México

2 Universidad Autónoma de Guerrero, Chilpancingo de los Bravo, México

*Address all correspondence to: manguzgm@gmail.com

† These authors contributed equally.

References

[1] Semenza JC, Menne B. Climate change and infectious diseases in Europe. Lancet ID. 2009;**9**:365-375. DOI: 10.1016/S1473-3099(09)70104-5

[2] World Health Organization [Internet]. 2020. Available from: https://www.who.int/news-room/fact-sheets/detail/vector-borne-diseases. [Accessed: 2022-03-23]

[3] Navarrete J, Vázquez J, Gómez H. Epidemiología del dengue y dengue hemorrágico en el Instituto Mexicano del Seguro Social (IMSS). Revista Peruana de Epidemiología. 2002; **10**(1):1-12

[4] Gaetan C, Guyon X. Second-order spatial models and geostatistics. In: Spatial Statistics and Modeling. Springer Series in Statistics. New York, NY: Springer; 2010. pp. 1-52. DOI: 10.1007/978-0-387-92257-7_1

[5] Hernández-Ávila JE, Rodríguez MH, Santos-Luna R, Sánchez-Castañeda V, Román-Pérez S, Ríos-Salgado VH, et al. Nation-wide, web-based, geographic information system for the integrated surveillance and control of dengue fever in Mexico. PLoS One. 2013;**8**(8):1-9. DOI: 10.1371/journal.pone.0070231

[6] Sinharay S. An overview of statistics in education. In: International Encyclopedia of Education. Third ed. Princeton, NJ, USA: Elsevier Science; 2011. pp. 1-11. DOI: 10.1016/B978-0-08-044894-7.01719-X

[7] Nelder JA, Wedderburn RWM. Generalized linear models. Journal of the Royal Statistical Society A. 1972;**135**: 370-384. DOI: 10.2307/2344614

[8] McCullagh P, Nelder JA. Generalized Linear Models. London, UK: Chapman and Hall; 1989

[9] Christensen OF, Waagepetersen R. Bayesian prediction of spatial count data using generalized linear mixed models. Biometrics. 2002;**58**(2):280-286

[10] Diggle P, Moyeed R, Rowlingson B, Thomson M. Childhood malaria in the Gambia: A case-study in model-based geostatistics. Journal of the Royal Statistical Society C. 2002;**51**(4):493-506

[11] Diggle PJ, Ribeiro PJ, Christensen OF. An introduction to model-based geostatistics. In: Møller J, editor. Spatial Statistics and Computational Methods. New York, NY, USA: Springer; 2003. pp. 43-86. DOI: 10.1007/978-0-387-21811-3_2

[12] Zhang H. On estimation and prediction for spatial generalized linear mixed models. Biometrics. 2002;**58**(1): 129-136. DOI: 10.1111/j.0006-341X.2002.00129.x

[13] Zhang H. Optimal interpolation and the appropriateness of cross-validating variogram in spatial generalized linear mixed models. Journal of Computational and Graphical Statistics. 2003;**12**(3): 698-713. DOI: 10.1198/1061860032265

[14] Saavedra A, Taboada J, Araújo M, Giráldez E. Generalized linear spatial models to predict slate exploitability. Journal of Applied Mathematics. 2013;**2013**:1-7. DOI: 10.1155/2013/531062

[15] Guyon X. Modelacion para la estadistica espacial. Revista de Investigacion Operacional. 2010;**31**(1): 1-33. DOI: 10.0257-4306

[16] Ver Hoef JM, Hanks EM, Hooten MB. On the relationship between conditional (CAR) and simultaneous

(SAR) autoregressive models. SpatStat. 2018;**25**:68-85

[17] Hashizume M, Dewan AM, Sunahara T, Rahman MZ, Yamamoto T. Hydroclimatological variability and dengue transmission in Dhaka, Bangladesh: A time-series study. BMC Infectious Diseases. 2012;**12**(98):1-9. DOI: 10.1186/1471-2334-12-98

[18] Breslow N, Clayton D. Approximate inference in generalized linear mixed models. Journal of the American Statistical Association. 1993;**88**:9-25. DOI: 10.2307/2290687

[19] Bandera Fernández E, Pérez PL. Los modelos lineales generalizados mixtos. Su aplicación en el mejoramiento de plantas. Cultivos Tropicales. 2018;**39**(1): 127-133. ISSN: 0258-5936

[20] Graham AJ, Atkinson PM, Danson FM. Spatial analysis for epidemiology. Science Direct. 2004;**91**(3):219-225. DOI: 10.1016/j.actatropica.2004.05.001

[21] Sánchez Pérez DL, Santa F, Fuentes López HJ. Spatial regression models for the behavior of infectious diseases dengue and malaria in Colombia for the years 2000, 2005 and 2010. Revista Geomática UD.GEO. 2012;**6**:110-128

[22] Estallo EL, Santana M, Martín ME, Galindo LM, Willener JA, Kuruc JA, et al. Environmental effects on phlebotominae sand flies (Diptera: Phychodidae) and implications for sand fly vector disease transmission in Corrientes city, northern Argentina. Anais da Academia Brasileira de Ciências. 2021;**93**(3):1-17. DOI: 10.1590/0001-3765202120191278

[23] Valbuena-Garcia AM, Rodríguez-Villamizar LA. Spatial analysis in epidemiology: Methodological review. Revista de la Universidad Industrial de Santander. Salud. 2018;**50**(4):358-365. DOI: 10.18273/revsal.v50n4-2018009

[24] Cressie N. Statistics for Spatial Data. Chichester-Toronto-Brisbane-Singapore. New York: John Wiley & Sons, Inc.; 1991. DOI: 10.1002/bimj.4710350210

[25] Sherman M. Spatial Statistics and Spatio-Temporal Data. Chichester, England: John Wiley & Sons, Inc; 2011. ISBN: 978-0-470-69958-4

[26] Chen Z, Wang B. How priors of initial hyperparameters affect Gaussian process regression models. Neurocomputing. 2018;**275**:1702-1710. DOI: 10.1016/j.neucom.2017.10.028

[27] Diggle PJ, Tawn JA, Moyeed RA. Model-based geostatistics. Journal of the Royal Statistical Society C. 1998;**47**(3): 299-350. DOI: 10.1111/1467-9876.00113

[28] Diggle PJ, Ribeiro PJ Jr. Model-based Geostatistics. In: Springer Series in Statistics. New York, NY, USA: Springer Science + Business Media, LLC; 2007. ISBN: 978-0-387-48536-2

[29] Gaetan C, Guyon X. Spatial Statistics and Modeling. New York: Springer; 2010. p. 90. ISBN: 9780387922577

[30] Kerry R, Oliver MA. Comparing sampling needs for variograms of soil properties computed by the method of moments and residual maximum likelihood. Geoderma. 2007;**140**(4): 383-396. DOI: 10.1016/j.geoderma.2007.04.019

[31] Diggle PJ, Tawn JA, Moyeed RA. Model-based geostatistics. Journal of the Royal Statistical Society: Series C (Applied Statistics). 1998;**47**(3):299-350. DOI: 10.1111/1467-9876.00113

[32] Moran PA. Notes on continuous stochastic phenomena. Biometrika. 1950; **37**(1/2):17-23. DOI: 10.2307/2332142

[33] Banerjee S, Carlin BP, Gelfand AE. Hierarchical Modeling and Analysis for Spatial Data. Florida, USA: CRC press; 2014. ISBN 9781439819173

[34] R Core Team. R: A Language and Environment for Statistical Computing. Vienna, Austria: R Foundation for Statistical Computing; 2021

[35] Ribeiro PJ Jr, Christensen OF, Diggle PJ. Geostatistical software - geoR and geoRglm. In: DSC 2003 Working Papers. Vienna, Austria: Distributed Statistical Computing; 2003

[36] Christensen OF, Ribeiro PJ. geoRglm: A Package for Generalised Linear Spatial Models. Vienna, Austria: R news; 2002

[37] Instituto Nacional de Estadística y Geografía. [Internet]. 2019. Available from: https://www.inegi.org.mx/. [Accessed: 2019-12-11]

[38] World Meteorological Organization [Internet]. 2019. Available from: https://public.wmo.int/es. [Accessed: 2019-11-23]

[39] Chan M, Johansson A. The incubation periods of dengue viruses. PLoS One. 2012;7(11):2-6. DOI: 10.1371/journal.pone.0050972

[40] Davison AC, Hinkley DV. Bootstrap Methods and their Application. Vol. No. 1. Cambridge, England: Cambridge University Press; 1997. DOI: 10.1017/CBO9780511802843

[41] Liu Z, Zhang Z, Lai Z, Zhou T, Jia Z, Gu J, et al. Temperature increase enhances Aedes albopictus competence to transmit dengue virus. Frontiers in Microbiology. 2017;**8**(2337):1-7. DOI: 10.3389/fmicb.2017.02337

[42] Aswi A, Cramb SM, Moraga P, Mengersen K. Bayesian spatial and spatio-temporal approaches to modelling dengue fever: A systematic review. Epidemiology and Infection. 2018; **29**(147):1-14

[43] Reinhold JM, Lazzari CR, Lahondère C. Effects of the environmental temperature on Aedes aegypti and Aedes albopictus mosquitoes: A review. Insects. 2018;**9** (4):1-17. DOI: 10.3390/insects9040158

[44] Phanitchat T, Zhao B, Haque U, et al. Spatial and temporal patterns of dengue incidence in northeastern Thailand 2006–2016. BMC Infectious Diseases. 2019;**19**(743):1-12. DOI: 10.1186/s12879-019-4379-3

Section 3

Clinical Trials

Chapter 8

Practical and Optimal Crossover Designs for Clinical Trials

Su Hwan Kim and Keumhee Chough Carriere

Abstract

Crossover designs have received great attention in clinical trials, as they allow subjects to serve as their own controls and gain such advantage as higher efficiency and smaller sample size over parallel designs, because the within-subject variability is in general smaller than between-subject variability. Response-adaptive crossover designs allow clinical trials to adapt and respond to the information acquired during the trials to achieve various objectives. Adaptive designs have been considered to allocate more subjects to superior treatments, improve statistical efficiency, reduce the sample size for cost savings, increase the sample size to maintain prespecified statistical power, or include auxiliary information. We focus on an adaptive allocation scheme to maximize the benefits from superior treatments, while maintaining a sufficiently high level of statistical efficiency, controlled by a suitable weight parameter. We review and discuss the strategy of incorporating multiple objectives, while advocating a regression type estimation approach via the Generalized Estimating Equations method. We show that the multiple objectives can be successfully incorporated to construct a spectrum of designs, ranging over various efficiencies and trial outcomes of success. Moreover, the adaptive allocation scheme successfully constructs designs with a desired efficiency, as illustrated by practical two- and three-period designs.

Keywords: crossover design, response adaptive allocation, optimal design, multiple objective function

1. Introduction

Crossover designs have enjoyed advantages over parallel designs, such as completely randomized design in terms of statistical efficiencies. Equal or balanced allocations play an important role in the construction of optimal designs under various model assumptions. However, equal allocations may pose ethical dilemma when researchers start to suspect that one treatment may be superior to the other. All trials start with the null hypothesis that the effects of a new treatment being tested are the same as comparators before we could prove its superiority. At some point in the trial, one may find an evidence indicating that the effects of treatments are notably different. Then, one may wonder whether to equally allocate remaining subjects to the treatments as per the protocol or to adapt to the findings and alter the allocation scheme to reflect the trial phenomena. Connor et al. [1] studied HIV treatment drug

IntechOpen

named AZT. Among 477 pregnant mothers with HIV, 239 were assigned to a placebo, and 238 were assigned to the AZT. The trial resulted in 60 infants diagnosed with HIV from the placebo group and 20 infants diagnosed with HIV from the AZT group. A decade later, Tymofyeyev et al. [2] suggested that use of 50–50 allocation was ethically improper given the seriousness of the outcome of the study and recommended to use a response-adaptive allocation. Tymofyeyev et al. [2] utilized the Play the Winner Rule (PWR) allocation [3, 4] and simulated the trial in a way that 360 and 117 pregnant mothers were adaptively allocated to the AZT or the placebo, respectively. The results of simulation showed that 60 infants were expected to be diagnosed with HIV in two groups combined as opposed to 80 infants in 1994, which revealed some of the benefits of the adaptive allocations.

Response-adaptive designs may have several other goals. Many authors [3–6] aimed at allocating more subjects to a better treatment. Armitage [7] aimed at reducing the sample size, and Wang [8] aimed at increasing the sample size based on the prespecified statistical power and the data acquired. Furthermore, Bandyopadhyay and Biswas [9] introduced covariates in response-adaptive designs. Sorkness et al. [10] proposed designs that were adaptive to the prevalence of events, in which the sample size recalculation was done to remedy the loss of statistical power arising from the imbalance of the prevalence. However, these studies utilized the acquired information using only a single objective. Many authors proposed a multiple objective adaptive design for continuous responses where they defined an objective function with two components, controlled by a weight parameter [11–13].

Binary responses are modeled differently from continuous responses in a way that the information is a function of the outcome. Standard logistic regression assumes that the responses are independent although crossover trial data are dependent on each subject. We use the Generalized Estimating Equations (GEEs) method, which can incorporate a desired covariance structure of responses. Liang and Zeger [14] proposed the GEE, which takes into account for the time dependencies of the data by allowing correlations. The GEE method estimates parameters by solving the system of equations based on the Quasi-Likelihood function. The advantage of Quasi-Likelihood method is that it does not need to provide joint distribution of the data and only requires the marginal distribution and its mean and variance. GEE estimates are proven consistent under a mild regularity conditions [14]. Valois [15] utilized GEE in the analysis of crossover designs.

This chapter demonstrates how to construct multiple objective response-adaptive designs for two treatments with binary outcomes using the GEE. We first review the theoretical grounds for crossover designs with binary outcome and the GEE method. Adaptive designs are constructed using simulations, and some two- and three-period practical designs will be built for various weights of multiple objective functions. We also compare the GEE methods to the other approaches done by Li [13]. Lastly, we develop a new strategy for maximizing the success outcome, while maintaining certain level of prefixed desired statistical efficiency.

2. Multiple objective response-adaptive designs with GEE

2.1 Model and information matrix

Agresti [16] discussed the Generalized Linear Model (GLM) for an exponential family of distributions. Suppose Y follows a distribution in an exponential family with parameters (θ, ϕ). Then the pdf of Y can be written as:

$$f(y|\theta, \phi) = \exp(y\theta - b(\theta))/a(\phi) + c(y, \phi)). \tag{1}$$

Consider that the Y_{ijk} denotes the binary response of ith period of jth subject in kth treatment sequence, distributed as Bernoulli (p_{ijk}), and X is a design matrix for an overall mean effect (μ), period effects (α_i), direct treatment effects ($\tau_{d(i,j,k)}$), and carryover effects ($\gamma_{d(i-1,j,k)}$) with the corresponding vector of parameters β. By defining the relation $\theta = h(\eta), \eta = x'\beta$ and with a logit link function $g()$, we can entertain the following model:

$$\eta_{ijk} = g(E(Y_{ijk})) = g(P(Y_{ijk} = 1) = \text{logit}(P(Y_{ijk} = 1)) \tag{2}$$

$$= \log\left(\frac{P(Y_{ijk} = 1)}{1 - P(Y_{ijk} = 1)}\right) = \mu + \alpha_i + \tau_{d(i,j,k)} + \gamma_{d(i-1,j,k)} = X'_{ijk}\beta_{ijk}. \tag{3}$$

It is easy to see that the mean and variance of Y_{ijk} are defined as

$$E(Y_{ijk}) = \mu_{ijk} = b'\left(\beta_{ijk}\right) = \frac{\exp\left(X'_{ijk}\beta_{ijk}\right)}{1 - \exp\left(X'_{ijk}\beta_{ijk}\right)}, \tag{4}$$

$$\text{Var}(Y_{ijk}) = \sigma_{ijk} = b''\left(\beta_{ijk}\right) = \frac{\exp\left(X'_{ijk}\beta_{ijk}\right)}{\left(1 - \exp\left(X'_{ijk}\beta_{ijk}\right)\right)^2}. \tag{5}$$

2.2 Generalized estimating equations

We use Generalized Estimating Equations to estimate the parameters of GLM with unknown correlation structure using the mean μ_{ijk} and unknown variance structure V_j^{-1}. The estimating equations can be shown as

$$\sum_{j=1}^{n} \frac{\partial \mu'_j}{\partial \beta} V_j^{-1}\left(Y_j - \mu_j\right) = 0, \tag{6}$$

where μ_j and Y_j are vector of means and responses for periods 1 to p.

The above estimating equation resembles that of GLM but does not require an exponential distribution assumption for Y, which is the strength of GEE. McCullaugh [17] showed that under the correct specification of mean and variance functions, the quasi-likelihood estimators demonstrate characteristics similar to MLE. The covariance matrix then can be written as:

$$\text{Var}(\beta) = \left[\sum_{j=1}^{n} \frac{\partial \mu'_j}{\partial \beta} V_j^{-1} \frac{\partial \mu_j}{\partial \beta}\right]^{-1} \tag{7}$$

Then, Bose and Dey [18] showed that the covariance matrix for parameters β can be defined with respect to k treatment sequences as follows:

$$\mathrm{Var}(\hat{\beta}) = \left(\sum_{k \in \Omega} n_k \frac{\partial \mu_k{}'}{\partial \beta} V_k^{-1} \frac{\partial \mu_k}{\partial \beta} \right)^{-1}, \tag{8}$$

where n_k denotes number of subjects allocated to kth sequence and the design matrices being identical for subjects in the same treatment sequence. However, when the specified covariance matrix V is not identical to the observed covariance matrix $\mathrm{Var}(Y)$, then the sandwich variance estimator is suggested:

$$\mathrm{Var}(\beta) = A \left(\sum_{k \in \Omega} n_k \frac{\partial \mu_j'}{\partial \beta} V_k^{-1} \mathrm{Var}(Y_k) V_k^{-1} \frac{\partial \mu_j}{\partial \beta} \right) A, \tag{9}$$

where A is the variance in Eq.(8). This sandwich variance estimator is shown to be consistent [14].

2.3 Multiple objective function

Liang and Carriere [11] proposed the following multiple objective function for the continuous responses:

$$\Phi_{j,k} = \lambda \frac{\Delta\left(\hat{I}_{j+1}^{k}(\beta)\right)}{\Delta\left(\hat{I}_{j+1}^{k'}(\beta)\right)} + (1-\lambda)\frac{f_{j,k}}{f_{j,k''}}, \tag{10}$$

where $\hat{I}_{j+1}^{k}(\beta)$ is the Fisher's Information matrix for subject $j+1$ allocated to treatment sequence k with Δ being an optimality criterion of choice and $f_{j,k}$ is an evaluation function for treatment sequence k based on the first j subjects in the trial. In this function, treatment sequence k' refers to the sequence with maximum $\hat{I}_{j+1}^{k}(\beta)$, and k'' refers to the sequence with maximum $f_{j,k}$, which may not necessarily be identical. Among the two terms in the objective function, the first term of the function investigates the efficiency of design with respect to the Fisher's information matrix given that subject $(j+1)$ is allocated to treatment sequence k. This is represented as a ratio over the sequence with maximum information so that the component may take value in $[0, 1]$. The second term of the function is called the evaluation function that evaluates the total efficacy of treatment sequences based on the estimated treatment effects. When $\lambda = 0$, the objective function considers only the efficiency of the design and ignores any superiority/inferiority of the treatments being tested. On the other hand, the objective function with $\lambda = 1$ would construct adaptive designs based solely on the positive effects of treatments being tested.

Liang et al. [12] and Li [13] extended their multiple objective function to binary responses and derived the information matrix for estimated success probabilities for binary responses. The observed number of successes for each treatment sequence was used for the evaluation function f. As the analysis of crossover trials mainly focuses on direct treatment effects, we choose the inverse of the variance of estimated treatment effects, $1/\mathrm{var}(\hat{\tau})$, as the criterion for comparing the efficiency of various treatment sequences. McCullagh [19] showed that quasi-likelihood estimates are invariant under a linear transformation. That is, $\hat{\mu}_k$ maximizes the quasi-likelihood function.

Throughout this chapter, we will refer to the Eq. (10) as the multiple objective function and choose the first term $\Delta\left(\hat{I}_{j+1}^{k}(\beta)\right)$ as the variance of the estimated treatment effects, $\text{var}\left(\hat{\tau}_{j+1,k}\right)$. The data acquired from the first j subjects are modeled using the GEE approach, and predictions for subject $j+1$ are made for all of the K treatment sequences. Then, we include the predicted responses of subject $j+1$ into the model and obtain the variance of an estimated treatment effects of each treatment sequence. Then, we evaluate the efficacy of each treatment sequence by using $\Sigma_{i=1}^{p}\hat{\eta}_{i,j,k}$. The $\eta's$ take any values in IR where large values correspond to a better treatment sequence. We transform these values to positive numbers so that a larger value indicates a better sequence and the ratios could be easily implemented. For this reason, we choose $f_{j,k} = \text{logit}\left(\Sigma_{i=1}^{p}\hat{\eta}_{i,j,k}\right)$, which falls in $(0,1)$ over all p periods.

3. Practical and nearly optimal designs

We apply the allocation method to construct some popular practical designs in clnical trials, two-treatment two-period designs and two-treatment three-period designs based on the parameter settings from Li [13], which are shown in **Table 1** with a slight modification on the values to incorporate the GEE modeling approach. Initially, one subject is assigned to each treatment sequence. Afterward, new subjects are introduced sequentially and are assigned to the treatment sequence with the highest Eq. (10). When all subjects are assigned, the variance of the estimated treatment effects, $\text{var}(\hat{\tau}_N)$, is computed and compared with the variance obtained from the optimal fixed designs suggested by Mukhopadhyay [20]. Mukhopadhyay [20] conducted simulation study for the optimal fixed crossover design with binary outcomes using the GEE method and showed that $AA/AB/BB/BA$ is optimal for $p = 2$ and

P	Parameters	Treatment sequences	Success probabilities	Expected success per period
2	$\mu = -0.22$	AA	$(0.60, 0.70)$	0.65
	$.\alpha_2 = 0.018$	AB	$(0.60, 0.40)$	0.50
	$.\tau = 0.63$	BA	$(0.30, 0.50)$	0.40
	$.\gamma = 0.42$	BB	$(0.30, 0.22)$	0.26
3	$\mu = -0.22$	AAA	$(0.60, 0.70, 0.65)$	0.65
	$.\alpha_2 = 0.018$	AAB	$(0.60, 0.70, 0.35)$	0.55
	$.\alpha_3 = -0.21$	ABA	$(0.60, 0.40, 0.44)$	0.48
	$.\tau = 0.63$	ABB	$(0.60, 0.40, 0.19)$	0.40
	$.\gamma = 0.4$	BAA	$(0.30, 0.50, 0.65)$	0.48
		BAB	$(0.30, 0.50, 0.35)$	0.38
		BBA	$(0.30, 0.22, 0.44)$	0.32
		BBB	$(0.30, 0.22, 0.19)$	0.23

Table 1.
Parameter values for simulation in construction of multiple-objective response-adaptive crossover design with binary outcomes.

$ABB/AAB/BAA/BBA$ is optimal for $p = 3$ under the compound symmetric covariance structure with binary outcomes.

3.1 Two-period design

There are four possible treatment sequences for two-treatment two-period crossover trials. Carriere and Reinsel [21] showed that an equal allocation on all sequences AA/BB/AB/BA, denoted as $d_{\text{opt},p2}$, is universally optimal for a continuous response, and Mukhopadhyay [20] confirmed that it is also numerically optimal even when responses are binary. We assign a subject to each of the four sequences and allocate the rest based on the objective function in Eq. (10). The following tables show the allocations of the adaptive designs, their efficiency compared with the fixed optimal design, and their success outcome ratio for various values of λ and N.

When $\lambda = 0$, the resulting allocation focuses on the treatment sequence AA with very few assigned to the rest of the sequences due to randomness during the initial stage of the trial. We can see that the allocation to the sequence AA decreases as λ increases. The allocations move toward a dual balanced design $d_{\text{opt},p2}$, which assigns equal allocations to all four sequences. The relative efficiency, which is defined as the ratio of variance of estimated treatment effects of $d_{\text{opt},p2}$ over the proposed multiple objective adaptive design, is low for $\lambda = 0$ and approaches 1 as λ increases to 1. The success ratio is close to the expected success shown in **Table 1** when $\lambda = 0$ and decreases as λ increases. Therefore, we must find a reasonable compromise between efficiency and a success ratio. For $n = 40$, $\lambda \in (0.85, 0.9)$ would construct an efficient design (efficiency > 0.8) with a sufficiently higher success ratio (5–8% increased) than $\lambda = 1$. For $n = 80$, $\lambda \in (0.9, 0.95)$ would construct a similar design (efficiency > 0.8 and success ratio improved by 5–8%). For $n = 100$, we note a drastic result around $\lambda \in (0.9, 0.95)$ where efficiency changes from 0.8957 to 0.7096, while the success ratio changes from 0.5168 to 0.5638, showing that the choice of suitable λ may vary significantly by the sample size n.

The consistent estimates for the above terms can be obtained by replacing the parameters with their GEE estimates. Also, the variance of the estimated β's can easily be computed using the sandwich covariance matrix from GEE. The treatment sequences with a smaller variance do not necessarily improve efficiency in this case, and the efficiency depends on the covariance matrix of the estimates of parameters. This covariance matrix, in turn, does not have a closed form, unlike in the continuous response case.

3.2 Three-period design

Three-period two-treatment crossover designs constructed from the multiple objective response-adaptive approach behave similarly as the two-period two-treatment designs. When $\lambda = 0$, the majority of the subjects are allocated to the treatment sequence AAA, which has the highest success ratio per period. For small sample size, $n = 40$, the efficiencies remain high and the success ratios are improved for any values of $\lambda < 1$. This is largely due to the conditions of the design, where $3 \times 8 = 24$ subjects out of 40 are assigned evenly to all eight sequences and thus only 16 subjects are allocated based on the multiple objective response-adaptive schemes. Therefore, the relative efficiency, which is computed based on the optimal design [20], remains high and the success ratio is improved only to a degree.

However, in the case of $n = 80$, the success ratio increases from 0.4323 to 0.5647 and the efficiency decreases from 1.0370 to 0.5793 as λ changes from 1 to 0. It is notable that the relative efficiencies of multiple objective response-adaptive designs for $\lambda = 1$ are greater than 1, indicating that these designs are slightly better than the optimal design [20] for the given set of parameters. The design with $\lambda = 0.95$ is as efficient as the optimal design, with a relative efficiency of 1.0055, and yet shows a higher success ratio (0.4708 compared with 0.4323), with an expected success ratio of 0.4696 (compared with 0.4375). In the case of $\lambda = 0.9$, the relative efficiency decreases to 0.9220 while the success ratio increases to 0.5050 from 0.4323. Looking at the design with $\lambda = 0.85$, we see that the relative efficiency decreases to 0.8133 while the success ratio increases to 0.5290. These two designs with $\lambda = 0.9$ and $\lambda = 0.85$ indicate that we could improve the success ratio of the design by 7–10% at the cost of relative efficiency between 0.1 and 0.2.

When $n = 100$, the designs show a similar performance to the case of $n = 80$ with respect to efficiency and the success ratio, except that efficiencies drop sharply, as we give attention to beneficial treatment effects with $\lambda < 1$.

In summary, the above tables show that adaptive schemes could benefit more subjects without much loss of efficiency for the given set of parameters. But it is important to find an appropriate λ to improve the success ratios while maintaining a sufficient level of statistical efficiency. In this case, $\lambda \in (0.85, 0.9)$ is recommended for both $n = 80$ and $n = 100$. However, we can see that the decrease in efficiency is more evident for $n = 100$ than that of $n = 80$, indicating that sample size N is another player determining the balance parameter λ. The resulting designs would have success ratios increased by 9–12% when compared with the optimal fixed design ($\lambda = 1$). Taking a smaller value of λ can benefit further, but the gain in success ratio decreases marginally as the λ decreases.

4. Comparison with other approaches

Bandyopadhyay [22] utilized an example of a three-period crossover trial of two treatments for hypertension. In this trial, 68 subjects were equally assigned to the treatment sequences $ABB/BAA/ABA/BAB$. Li [13] used the last two periods of this trial to obtain a crossover design with $AA/BB/AB/BA$. The response variable was continuous measurements of systolic blood pressure. Binary response variables were computed by dichotomizing the blood pressures at "135 or more" and "140 or more" and denoting the responses as failures. Two corresponding sets of success probabilities were estimated from this data. $(\hat{v}_{A1}, \hat{v}_{A2}, \hat{v}_{B1}, \hat{v}_{B2}) = (0.24, 0.24, 0.24, 0.35)$ and $(\hat{v}_{A1}, \hat{v}_{A2}, \hat{v}_{B1}, \hat{v}_{B2}) = (0.35, 0.5, 0.35, 0.53)$ where v is the probability of success with the letters denoting treatments and numbers denoting periods.

These estimated probabilities were considered as actual success probabilities, and the multiple objective response-adaptive technique was applied with $\lambda = 1$ and $\lambda = 0.9$. A comparison of allocations, efficiencies, and success ratios of the three methods (B, L, K proposed by [13, 20, 23], respectively) is provided below. We included fixed group effects, β_k, to the model in Eq. (2) to incorporate success probabilities. The parameters and other settings are provided in **Table 2**, and the results of simulations are found in **Tables 3** and **4**.

The efficiencies in **Table 3** were computed against the equal allocation design, which are nonadaptive but optimal for two-period and two-treatment designs. First, we examine multiple objective response-adaptive designs with $\lambda = 1$. We see that when the

Probabilities	Parameters	Treatment sequences	Success probabilities	Expected success per period
$\hat{v}_{A1} = 0.24$	$\mu = -1.89, \beta_1 = 1$	AA	$(0.24, 0.24)$	0.240
$\hat{v}_{A2} = 0.24$	$\alpha_2 = 0.27, \beta_2 = 1$	AB	$(0.24, 0.35)$	0.295
$\hat{v}_{B1} = 0.24$	$\tau = -0.27, \beta_3 = 0.47$	BA	$(0.24, 0.24)$	0.240
$\hat{v}_{B2} = 0.35$	$\gamma = -0.27, \beta_4 = 0.47$	BB	$(0.24, 0.35)$	0.295
$\hat{v}_{A1} = 0.35$	$\mu = -1.56, \beta_1 = 1$	AA	$(0.35, 0.50)$	0.425
$\hat{v}_{A2} = 0.5$	$\alpha_2 = 0.68, \beta_2 = 1$	AB	$(0.35, 0.53)$	0.440
$\hat{v}_{B1} = 0.35$	$\tau = -0.06, \beta_3 = 0.88$	BA	$(0.35, 0.50)$	0.425
$\hat{v}_{B2} = 0.53$	$\gamma = -0.06, \beta_4 = 0.88$	BB	$(0.35, 0.53)$	0.440

Table 2.
Parameter values and expected success probabilities based on the crossover trial of [22].

Parameters	Design	λ	AA	AB	BA	BB	Efficiency	Expected success
$(\hat{v}_{A1}, \hat{v}_{A2}, \hat{v}_{B1}, \hat{v}_{B2})$ (0.24, 0.24, 0.24, 0.35)	d_1^B		15.75	16.92	17.01	18.32	0.9912	0.2685
	d_2^L	1	13.13	21.03	13.03	20.80	0.9143	0.2738
	d_3^L	0.1	14.69	19.06	13.64	20.62	0.9522	0.2729
	d_4^K	1	12.81	20.85	12.49	21.85	0.8913	0.2745
	d_5^K	0.1	15.22	19.58	14.19	19.01	0.9829	0.2713
	d_6^E		17.00	17.00	17.00	17.00	1.0000	0.2675
(0.35, 0.50, 0.35, 0.53)	d_7^B		13.00	16.42	16.46	22.12	0.9769	0.4335
	d_8^L	1	7.32	16.35	14.88	29.46	0.8376	0.4352
	d_9^L	0.1	12.38	16.71	15.80	23.11	0.9627	0.4338
	d_{10}^K	1	16.22	17.89	15.40	18.49	0.9970	0.4330
	d_{11}^K	0.1	16.76	17.53	16.80	16.91	0.9983	0.4326
	d_6^E		17.00	17.00	17.00	17.00	1.0000	0.4325

[B] [22]; [L] [13]; [K] [23]; [E] Equal allocation design.

Table 3.
Allocation, efficiency, and success ratio for two-period designs.

difference of the expected success probabilities between the sequences is small (0.425 vs. 0.44, second example in **Table 2**), [13]'s strategy allocates an extensive number of the subjects to the treatment sequences AB/BB and results in a substantial loss of efficiency. Moreover, the gain in the expected success over an equal allocation design is minimal (0.4352 vs. 0.4325). The simulations confirm this observation, and d_8 has relative efficiency of 0.8376 without much gain as a result. On the other hand, d_{10} adapts to the small differences in the sequences in a careful manner, and it assigns about three more subjects to better treatment sequences AB/BB without losing efficiency (0.9970). d_{10} allocates fewer subjects to AB/BB compared with d_7, d_8, and d_9.

It is noticeable that the pattern is not the same when there is some difference in the expected success probabilities between the treatment sequences (0.24 vs. 0.295). Design d_2 allocates 41.83 subjects to better sequences AB/BB, whereas d_4 allocates 42.7

N	Designs	AA	AB	BA	BB	Efficiency	Success ratio
40	$d_{(0.8)}$	22.22	7.60	5.63	4.55	0.7615	0.5420
	$d_{(0.9)}$	16.63	9.49	7.28	6.60	0.9152	0.5042
	$d_{(1)}$	10.20	10.01	9.66	10.13	1.0141	0.4534
	$d_{Adaptive}$	21.75	6.11	6.21	5.94	0.8465	0.5319
80	$d_{(0.9)}$	45.08	16.64	10.56	7.72	0.7582	0.5507
	$d_{(0.95)}$	33.68	18.98	13.95	13.39	0.9368	0.5048
	$d_{(1)}$	20.35	19.81	18.96	20.88	1.0076	0.4532
	$d_{Adaptive}$	43.58	12.35	12.24	11.83	0.8430	0.5309
100	$d_{(0.9)}$	61.75	19.36	11.01	7.89	0.7096	0.5638
	$d_{(0.95)}$	45.77	23.49	16.30	14.44	0.8957	0.5168
	$d_{(1)}$	25.41	24.40	23.66	26.54	1.0258	0.4525
	$d_{Adaptive}$	57.09	14.42	14.12	14.37	0.7972	0.5391

Table 4.
Comparison of new revised response-adaptive two-period design with the results from ***Table** 5.*

subjects. The designs allocate more subjects to better treatment sequences than d_1 while maintaining a high level of efficiency.

The designs constructed using the multiple objective response-adaptive method with GEE are more responsive to the differences in treatments better than Bandyopadhyay [22] and Li [13], while maintaining a high level of efficiency when there is a large difference in the treatment effects. The method by Kim [23] assigns more subjects to the better treatment sequence when the treatment differences are large. Moreover, the resulting designs are close to the optimal design with an equal allocations on all four sequences, when the treatment differences are negligible. This assures that even if the treatment difference is not as large as expected, the multiple objective response-adaptive method is robust and creates an efficient design.

5. Implementing the adaptive allocations

In **Tables 5** and **6**, we observed that the decrease in efficiency following the decrease in λ is not consistent for differing sample sizes. That is, if we wish to maintain some level of relative efficiency with respect to a known fixed optimal design while applying the multiple objective adaptive allocation scheme, we must fully understand the behaviors of this adaptive allocation scheme and find the suitable λ, which is determined by the true parameters as well as the sample size. The simulations on this scheme may help suggest some λ's, but is limited to the specific scenarios being studied. Therefore, we implement a sensible strategy of the multiple-objective-based allocation scheme without having to precisely know which λ to use.

The multiple-objective function as in Eq. (10) is now split into two objective functions:

$$H_{1,j,k} = \frac{\Delta\left(\hat{I}^{k}_{j+1}(\beta)\right)}{\Delta\left(\hat{I}^{k'}_{j+1}(\beta)\right)}, \tag{11}$$

N	λ	AA	AB	BA	BB	Efficiency	Success ratio
40	0	26.97	4.37	4.51	4.15	0.5679	0.5635
	0.3	26.46	4.40	4.94	4.20	0.5696	0.5596
	0.7	25.42	5.46	4.89	4.23	0.6378	0.5576
	0.8	22.22	7.60	5.63	4.55	0.7615	0.5420
	0.9	16.63	9.49	7.28	6.60	0.9152	0.5042
	1	10.20	10.01	9.66	10.13	1.0141	0.4534
80	0	65.81	4.53	5.46	4.20	0.2998	0.6046
	0.3	66.05	4.65	5.13	4.17	0.3012	0.6055
	0.7	64.37	5.95	5.43	4.26	0.3554	0.6020
	0.8	59.16	9.95	6.28	4.60	0.4844	0.5896
	0.9	45.08	16.64	10.56	7.72	0.7582	0.5507
	0.95	33.68	18.98	13.95	13.39	0.9368	0.5048
	1	20.35	19.81	18.96	20.88	1.0076	0.4532
100	0	85.14	4.71	5.85	4.31	0.2859	0.6126
	0.3	85.84	4.56	5.45	4.15	0.2773	0.6136
	0.7	84.57	6.03	5.25	4.16	0.3184	0.6114
	0.9	61.75	19.36	11.01	7.89	0.7096	0.5638
	0.95	45.77	23.49	16.30	14.44	0.8957	0.5168
	1	25.41	24.40	23.66	26.54	1.0258	0.4525

Table 5.
Allocation, efficiency, and success ratio for two-period designs using the multiple objective criteria in Eq. (10).

$$H_{2,j,k} = \frac{f_{j,k}}{f_{j,k''}}, \tag{12}$$

which are the first and second terms of the Eq. (10). The allocation scheme takes the following steps.

1. Determine a desirable relative efficiency r^*, e.g., 80%.

2. Acquire a small number of subjects to each sequence and obtain the quasi-likelihood estimates of the parameters, μ, π_i's, τ, γ from a logistic model.

3. Generate another set of data with the same number of total subjects as the current dataset with allocations according to the optimal design $d_{\text{opt},p2}$. Obtain estimates of the parameters and sandwich covariance matrices of the estimated parameters from the new data and compare the efficiencies of two designs, $r = \text{var}(\hat{\tau}_{\text{opt}})/\text{var}(\hat{\tau}_{\text{Adaptive}})$.

4. If $r < r^*$, then use $H_{1,j,k}$ as the allocation function for subject $j+1$, otherwise use $H_{2,j,k}$ as the allocation function for subject $j+1$.

5. Return to step 2 until all subjects are allocated.

N	λ	AAA	AAB	ABA	ABB	BAA	BAB	BBA	BBB	Efficiency	Success ratio
40	0	11.98	4.00	4.01	4.00	4.00	4.00	4.01	4.00	0.9603	0.4797
	0.3	11.95	4.02	4.00	4.00	4.01	4.00	4.02	4.00	0.9631	0.4785
	0.7	10.97	4.77	4.12	4.12	4.11	4.01	4.00	4.00	0.9891	0.4767
	0.8	9.24	5.62	4.73	4.56	5.01	4.55	4.36	4.23	0.9931	0.4678
	0.9	6.94	5.62	4.73	4.56	5.01	4.55	4.36	4.23	1.0075	0.4566
	1	5.04	5.03	4.73	4.96	4.98	4.93	4.97	5.36	1.0302	0.4377
80	0	51.98	4.01	4.00	4.00	4.00	4.00	4.01	4.00	0.5793	0.5647
	0.3	51.95	4.00	4.01	4.00	4.01	4.00	4.00	4.00	0.5848	0.5656
	0.7	49.58	5.91	4.24	4.01	4.23	4.01	4.02	4.00	0.6043	0.5619
	0.8	41.09	10.41	6.07	4.24	5.89	4.24	4.06	4.00	0.7223	0.5458
	0.85	33.85	12.40	7.48	5.14	7.47	5.20	4.39	4.07	0.8133	0.5290
	0.9	25.20	13.16	8.67	6.74	9.10	6.94	5.63	4.56	0.9220	0.5050
	0.95	16.76	12.06	9.02	8.48	10.27	8.61	7.94	6.86	1.0055	0.4708
	1	10.09	9.97	8.58	9.95	9.83	9.75	9.91	11.92	1.0370	0.4323
100	0	71.97	4.01	4.00	4.00	4.00	4.00	4.02	4.00	0.4972	0.5817
	0.3	71.98	4.01	4.00	4.00	4.01	4.00	4.00	4.01	0.5081	0.5805
	0.7	69.41	6.03	4.28	4.02	4.25	4.01	4.00	4.00	0.5379	0.5812
	0.8	57.12	6.09	5.56	6.20	6.01	5.95	6.18	6.90	0.6345	0.5445
	0.85	54.13	12.65	7.646	4.94	7.32	5.00	4.28	4.05	0.6951	0.5553
	0.9	37.37	16.65	10.20	7.39	10.46	7.62	5.80	4.50	0.8696	0.5231
	0.95	23.93	15.91	10.85	10.17	12.35	10.44	9.17	7.19	0.9858	0.4794
	1	12.45	12.50	10.38	12.57	12.10	12.18	12.49	15.32	1.0435	0.4315

Table 6.
Allocation, efficiency, and success ratio for three-period design using the multiple objective criteria in Eq. (10).

To illustrate, we apply the above strategy to the parameters in **Table 1** with the aim of constructing a response-adaptive design with a relative efficiency around $r^* > 0.8$. First, we construct two-period two-treatment response-adaptive designs with $n = 40$, 80, and 100. We present the results for three-period two-treatment designs with $n = 80$ and 100. The case for $n = 40$ was excluded as all adaptive designs constructed using Eq. (10) with any λ have relative efficiencies > 0.9.

From **Table 4**, we can see that the designs constructed using the adaptive allocation method by Kim [23], denoted as d_{Adaptive}, have relative efficiencies close to 0.8 or slightly larger than that while the success ratios are increased by 9% compared with the designs for $\lambda = 1$. For $n = 40$, the adaptive design follows the pattern of changes in the allocations, efficiency, and success ratio so that we can find one between $d_{(0.8)}$ and $d_{(0.9)}$. For example, the allocation to the treatment sequence *AA* is 21.75 (d_{Adaptive}), which is between 16.63 ($d_{(0.8)}$) and 22.22 ($d_{(0.9)}$). This pattern is also the case for all other columns in the table for $n = 80$ and 100. Our adaptive designs appear to be constructed in a similar manner as the multiple objective response-adaptive designs as if they were constructed with the λ in the suggested range of

N	Designs	AAA	AAB	ABA	ABB	BAA	BAB	BBA	BBB	Efficiency	Success ratio
80	$d_{(0.8)}$	41.09	10.41	6.07	4.24	5.89	4.24	4.06	4.00	0.7223	0.5458
	$d_{(0.9)}$	25.20	13.16	8.67	6.74	9.10	6.94	5.63	4.56	0.9220	0.5050
	$d_{(0.95)}$	16.76	12.06	9.02	8.48	10.27	8.61	7.94	6.86	1.0055	0.4708
	$d_{(1)}$	10.09	9.97	8.58	9.95	9.83	9.75	9.91	11.92	1.0370	0.4323
	$d_{Adaptive}$	39.49	5.25	7.35	5.42	4.98	5.02	6.88	5.61	0.7999	0.5267
100	$d_{(0.7)}$	69.41	6.03	4.28	4.02	4.25	4.01	4.00	4.00	0.5379	0.5812
	$d_{(0.8)}$	57.12	6.09	5.56	6.20	6.01	5.95	6.18	6.90	0.6345	0.5445
	$d_{(0.9)}$	37.37	16.65	10.20	7.39	10.46	7.62	5.80	4.50	0.8696	0.5231
	$d_{(0.95)}$	23.93	15.91	10.85	10.17	12.35	10.44	9.17	7.19	0.9858	0.4794
	$d_{(1)}$	12.45	12.50	10.38	12.57	12.10	12.18	12.49	15.32	1.0435	0.4315
	$d_{Adaptive}$	50.48	5.93	9.52	6.45	5.65	5.78	9.11	7.08	0.7854	0.5278

Table 7.
Comparison of our new revised response-adaptive three-period design with the results from ***Table 6****.*

$(0.8, 0.9)$. Similarly, the d_{Adaptive} designs for $n = 80$ and $n = 100$ fall right in between $d_{(0.9)}$ and $d_{(0.95)}$.

From **Table 7**, the relative efficiencies of our adaptive three-period designs are 0.7999 and 0.7854 for $n = 80$ and $n = 100$, respectively. These efficiencies are very close to our target $r^* = 0.8$ while the success ratios are improved by approximately 9%. We can see that the allocation for treatment sequence AAA, relative efficiency, and the success ratio for the new adaptive designs d_{Adaptive} follow the same pattern as the multiple objective response-adaptive designs. The allocations to the other sequences are relatively small and do not seem to affect the efficiency much as long as the allocation to AAA is well controlled. The above strategy successfully leads us to obtain desired success ratios and maintain efficiency to a prespecified level without having to determine what the ideal λ is.

6. Conclusion

This chapter discussed practical and nearly optimal designs for clinical trials. One of the major concerns is that response-adaptive designs have so much potential to complement the traditional experimental designs. The use of the data acquired during the trial may benefit the trial in numerous ways such as improving the statistical power, reducing the cost of the trial by recalculating the required sample size, assigning more subjects to a better treatment or treatment sequences, or utilizing the information acquired from the covariates to improve efficiency. The multiple objective criteria may incorporate more components or select various other sets of components such as cost efficiency versus statistical efficiency and many others.

To achieve any efficiency in trials with binary responses, we start by recognizing that they have distinct properties that are different from continuous responses in that their means and variances are functions of the outcomes. As a result, binary response designs are response-dependent. Due to this characteristic, the construction of optimal designs for binary responses requires special attention. Due in part to these difficulty, there are limited studies on response-adaptive designs and optimal designs in the literature for binary outcome data. In this chapter, we compared approaches of constructing response-adaptive designs. Also, we conducted a simulation study based on an actual data example to investigate the performance of the multiple objective response-adaptive designs using the GEE over the other two methods.

We demonstrated by constructing response-adaptive designs using an objective function, namely the multiple objective function. The designs constructed using the multiple objective function were highly efficient, successful with respect to desirable or beneficial treatment outcomes. In **Tables 5** and **6**, we observed that the choice of λ for an efficient and successful design would depend on the sample size and the true values of μ, $\pi_i's$, τ, and γ. The efficiencies drop significantly when n increases or λ decreases. These designs may have significantly higher success ratios but may also have significantly low efficiency (<0.6), which is undesirable.

We then compared the approach by Kim [23] to other multiple objective adaptive designs using the GEE to the response-adaptive design by Mukhopadhyay [20] and multiple objective adaptive designs using binary probability modeling approach by Li [13] for two-period two-treatment crossover designs. The proposed designs responded to the differences in the treatment effects in a rather robust manner. When the treatment difference is very small, the proposed designs were very close to the optimal design with an equal allocation on four treatment sequences, $AA/AB/BA/BB$, as expected. On the other hand, the other two methods assign too large a proportion of subjects to treatment sequences BB and lose efficiencies for very small gain in successful outcome ratios. When the treatment difference is large, the design with $\lambda = 1$ assigns more subjects to a better treatment sequences compared with the other two designs considered by Bandyopadhyay et al. [5] and Li [13].

We observed that the choice of λ was very important in finding a balance between the relative efficiency and a success ratio. One may suggest some appropriate range of λ, but it is valid for only a certain set of parameters and sample size, and the true parameters are usually unknown. To overcome this challenge, Kim [23] devised a multiple objective response-adaptive scheme, which utilizes all of the two components of Eq. (10), not simultaneously but in a sequential manner. The simulation results show that this adaptive scheme can construct designs with desired relative ratios without having to select the weight parameter λ. The scheme by Kim [23] allows researchers to run an adaptive trial knowing that their design would find the balance between two important components of the trial—statistically efficiency and higher allocation to a beneficial treatment.

Author details

Su Hwan Kim and Keumhee Chough Carriere*
Department of Mathematical and Statistical Sciences, University of Alberta, Edmonton, AB, Canada

*Address all correspondence to: kccarrie@ualberta.ca

References

[1] Connor EM, Sperling RS, Gelber R, Kiselev P, Scott G, O'Sullivan MJ, et al. Reduction of maternal-infant transmission of human immunodeficiency virus type 1 with zidovudine treatment. New England Journal of Medicine. 1994; **331**:1173-1180

[2] Tymofyeyev Y, Rosenberger WF, Hu F. Implementing optimal allocation in sequential binary response experiments. Journal of the American Statistical Association. 2007;**102**(477): 224-234

[3] Zelen M. Play the winner rule and the controlled clinical trial. Journal of American Statistical Association. 2003; **64**:131-146

[4] Wei LJ, Durham S. The randomized play-the-winner rule in medical trials. Journal of American Statistical Association. 1978;**73**:840-843

[5] Bandyopadhyay U, Biswas A, Mukherjee S. Randomized play-the-winner rule in two-period two-treatment repeated measurement design. Austrian Journal of Statistics. 2009;**38**:151-169

[6] Bandyopadhyay U, Biswas A, Mukherjee S. Adaptive two-treatment two-period crossover design for binary treatment responses incorporating carry-over effects. Statistical Methods and Applications. 2009;**18**:13-33

[7] Armitage P. Sequential Medical Trials. Oxford: Blackwell; 1975

[8] Wang J. Adaptive Optimal Two Treatment Crossover Designs with Binary Endpoint. Chicago: University of Illinois; 2014

[9] Bandyopadhyay U, Biswas A. Adaptive designs for normal responses with prognostic factors. Biometrika. 2001;**88**:409-419

[10] Sorkness CA, King TS, Dyer AM, Chinchilli VM, Mauger DT, Krishnan JA, et al. Adapting clinical trial design to maintain meaningful outcomes during a multicenter asthma trial in the precision medicine era. Contemporary Clinical Trials. 2019;**77**:98-103

[11] Liang Y, Carriere KC. Multiple-objective response-adaptive repeated measurement designs for clinical trials. Journal of Statistical Planning and Inference. 2009;**139**:1134-1145

[12] Liang Y, Li Y, Wang J, Carriere KC. Multiple-objective response-adaptive repeated measurement designs in clinical trials for binary responses. Statistics in Medicine. 2014;**33**(4): 607-617

[13] Li Y. Optimal Crossover Designs in Clinical Trials., PhD dissertation. University of Alberta; 2017

[14] Liang KY, Zeger S. Longitudinal data analysis using generalized linear models. Biometrika. 1986;**73**(1):13-22

[15] Valois MF. Evaluation of the Performance of the Generalized Estimating Equations Method for the Analysis of Crossover Design. Montreal: McGill University; 1997

[16] Agresti A. Categorical Data Analysis. Hoboken: Wiley; 2014

[17] McCullagh P. Generalized Linear Models. Boca Raton: Chapman and Hall/ CRC; 1999

[18] Bose M, Dey A. Optimal Crossover Designs. New Jersey: World Scientic; 2009

[19] McCullagh P. Quasi-Likelihood Functions. The Annals of Statistics. 2005;**11**(1):59-67

[20] Mukhopadhyay S. Optimal Two-Treatment Crossover Designs for Binary Response Models. Cornell University system. arXiv:1505.02488, 2015

[21] Carriere KC, Reinsel GC. Optimal two-period repeated measurement designs with two or more treatments. Biometrika. 1993;**80**(4):924-929

[22] Bandyopadhyay U, Biswas A, Mukherjee S. Adaptive two-treatment two-period crossover design for binary treatment responses. Statistica Neerlandica. 2007;**61**(3):329-334

[23] Kim SH. Practical and Optimal Crossover Designs for Clinical Trials. Ph.D. dissertation. University of Alberta; 2019

Chapter 9

Optimal N-of-1 Clinical Trials for Individualized Patient Care and Aggregated N-of-1 Designs

Yin Li, Weng Kee Wong and Keumhee Chough Carriere

Abstract

Precision medicine typically refers to the use of genomic signatures of patients to assign more effective therapies to treat patients, or, for improved diagnosis of the early onset of a disease so that interventions can be delivered to prevent or delay the disease progression. Because the aim is to provide individualized patient treatment, such single-person trials are called N-of-1 trials. This chapter reviews fundamental ideas, models, and construction of optimal designs for N-of-1 trials, which are invariably constructed from crossover trials, where each patient receives a random sequence of trial treatments over time. We construct examples of universally optimal N-of-1 designs for comparing two treatments under various correlation structure assumptions and discuss how N-of-1 trials may be combined to form optimal aggregated N-of-1 trials for assessing average treatment effects for two or more treatments.

Keywords: crossover design, individualized care, N-of-1 trials, precision medicine, universally optimal designs

1. Introduction

N-of-1 trials or single-patient trials focus on one patient and their main goal is to evaluate whether the treatment is effective for the individual. The main motivation for such trials is that each patient serves as his or her own control, and another is that each patient is different from another and there is no average patient. This is in contrast to conventional clinical trials where the aim is to optimize treatment for the average patients. Consequently, their aims are different, and conventional clinical trials are not appropriate for N-of-1 trials. These trials may appear new but they are not, except that they probably were given short shrift and not well publicized. In the last decade or so, there is increasing interest in N-of-1 trials. Duan et al. [1] raised awareness among clinicians and epidemiologists that N-of-1 trials are potentially useful for informing personalized treatment decisions for patients with chronic conditions. A monograph on this topic in healthcare is [2], where their applications to behavioral sciences and many medical settings are discussed, including the economics, ethics, statistical analysis of running such trials, and how to report results to professional audiences. Scuffham et al. [3] showed how N-of-1 trials can improve patient management and save costs and Kravitz and Duan [4] provided a user's handbook on implementing such trials. A systematic review of the use of N-of-1 trials in the medical literature is given in [5]. There are many ways to analyze and compare results from N-of-1 trials; see for example, [6].

Interestingly, and perhaps, not unexpectedly, results from N-of-1 trials can be combined to generate group mean effects, as [7, 8] demonstrated how it can be done using systematic reviews and meta-analyses on the effects of amphetamine and methylphenidate for attention-deficit hyperactivity disorder. Li et al. [9] provided a systematic review of quality N-of-1 trials published between 1985 and 2013 in the medical literature based on the CONSORT extension for N-of-1 Trials (CENT) where they examined factors that influence reporting quality in these trials. In palliative care, Senior et al. [10] designed a N-of-1 trial of a psychostimulant, methylphenidate hydrochloride (MPH) (5 mg bd), compared to placebo as a treatment for fatigue, with a population estimate of the benefit by the aggregation of multiple SPTs. Forty patients who had advanced cancer was enrolled through specialist palliative care services in Australia.

Multi-crossover single-patient trials are often employed when the focus is to make the best possible treatment decision for an individual patient [2, 11, 12]. From a clinician's perspective, having clear evidence of the value of one treatment over another (or no treatment) is more useful than knowing the average response. The average response gives the clinician the probability that a treatment will be effective, whereas N-of-1 trials give more certainty about whether the treatment for a particular patient will work or not.

In what is to follow, we assume that there are predetermined p periods in the crossover study, and in each period only one of the treatments is administrated. The same treatment may be used in other periods. We first discuss the case when there are two treatments and two periods for N-of-1 trials before extending them to aggregated N-of-1 trials to evaluate the effects of treatments for the average patients. Treatment groups are generically denoted by *A*, *B*, *C*, and so on.

Many researchers studied the optimality of crossover designs [13–18]. Optimal designs have been constructed under a variety of statistical models to provide the most accurate inference of the treatment effects. It is known that the two-treatment design *AB*, *AA* and their duals *BA*, *BB* are found to be universally optimal for two-period experiments, with the duality defined as the sequence that switches *A* and *B* with the same effect. Similarly, it is known that the two-sequence design *ABB* and its dual *BAA* and the four-sequence design *ABBA*, *AABB* and their duals *BAAB*, *BBAA* are optimal for three- and four-period experiments, respectively [19] and [20].

A direct application of this two-treatment optimal design results from the literature with *A* replaced as *AB* and *B* as *BA* would suggest that optimal N-of-1 trials can use the four-sequence design with *ABBA*, *ABAB* or their duals for two within-patient comparisons. Similarly, the two-sequence design with *ABBABA* or its dual may be optimal for three within-patient comparisons, and the four-sequence design with *ABBABAAB*, *ABABBABA* or any of their duals may be optimal for four within-patient comparisons.

However, design issues are not always as straightforward to address. For example, Carriere and Li [21] showed that constructing N-of-1 trials for individualized care from sequences in these repeated measurement designs is not always optimal for estimating individual-based treatment effects. Likewise, Guyatt et al. [22] showed that aggregating a series of N-of-1 trials that are optimal for individual patients can also provide an optimal estimate of the treatment effects for the average patient. For example, in a multi-clinic setting in three *AB* pair six-period N-of-1 studies, all eight possible sequences ($2^{6/2} = 8$) have been used, i.e., *ABABAB*, *ABABBA*, *ABBAAB*, *ABBABA* and their duals to estimate both individual-based and average treatment effects. However, we show how these do not lead to optimal aggregated N-of-1 trials for estimating the treatment effects for the average patient.

2. Models and information matrix

The traditional crossover design model assumes that the carryover effects last for only one period. The patient effects are considered fixed in the model. The traditional model assumes no carryover effects for the observations in the first period. An alternative model which has carryover effects in the first period as well is built by giving patients a pre-period or baseline period [23, 24]. More complex models have also been considered. Some models incorporate higher-order carryover effects [25]; some consider carryover effects are proportional to the treatment effects [26], some include the interaction effects between the treatment effects and carryover effects [27], and others have random patient effects [28–30].

We first focus on the traditional model, frequently used to analyze repeated measures crossover data:

$$Y_{ij} = \mu + \alpha_i + \beta_j + \tau_{d(i,j)} + \gamma_{d(i-1,j)} + \varepsilon_{ij}, \tag{1}$$

$i = 1, \cdots, p$ and $j = 1, \cdots, N$. Here Y_{ij} is the outcome in the ith period from the jth patient; α_i is the ith period effect and β_j is the jth patient effect. Further, $d(i,j)$ represents the treatment assigned to the patient in period i of patient j, and $\tau_{d(i,j)}$ and $\gamma_{d(i-1,j)}$ are, respectively, the treatment effect of the treatment in the ith period and the carryover effect of the treatment in the $(i-1)^{th}$ period.

The model assumes that the carryover effects only depend on the treatment assigned in the previous period but not on the treatment in the current period, which may be unrealistic. Taking the interaction into account without introducing too many parameters, Kunert and Stufken [17] presented a model with self and mixed carryover effects. The self carryover effect occurs when the treatments administered in the current and the previous periods are the same; otherwise, we have a mixed carryover effect. The model with the self and mixed carryover effects is given by

$$Y_{ij} = \begin{cases} \mu + \alpha_i + \beta_j + \tau_{d(i,j)} + \gamma_{s,d(i-1,j)} + \varepsilon_{ij}, & \text{if d(i, j) = d(i-1, j)} \\ \mu + \alpha_i + \beta_j + \tau_{d(i,j)} + \gamma_{m,d(i-1,j)} + \varepsilon_{ij}, & \text{if d(i, j)} \neq \text{d(i-1, j)} \end{cases}, \tag{2}$$

where α_i, β_j, $d(i,j)$ and $\tau_{d(i,j)}$, are defined as in model (1). The parameters $\gamma_{s,d(i-1,j)}$ and $\gamma_{m,d(i-1,j)}$ represent the self and mixed carryover effects of the treatment assigned in the $(i-1)^{th}$ period, respectively.

In an N-of-1 trial with $N = 1$, the j index can be omitted. Further, with one patient and p responses in total, the period effects and patient effects cannot be accommodated. Therefore, we need to reduce the models for the case when $N = 1$.

For models (1) and (2), we define the contrast of the direct treatment effects by $\tau = (\tau_A - \tau_B)/2$, the contrast of the first-order carryover effects by $\gamma = (\gamma_A - \gamma_B)/2$, the contrast of the self carryover effects by $\gamma_s = (\gamma_{s,A} - \gamma_{s,B})/2$ and the contrast of the mixed carryover effects by $\gamma_m = (\gamma_{m,A} - \gamma_{m,B})/2$.

To construct a model-based optimal design, we commonly use design criteria such as A-, D-, and E-optimality. The A-, D-, and E-optimal design maximizes the trace, the determinant, or the eigenvalue of the information matrix among a class of all competing designs. The information matrix measures the amount of information about the unknown model parameters. Formally, given the model and the design, the elements in the information matrix are found by first taking the expectation of the second derivatives of the complete log-likelihood function with respect to the parameters and multiplying them by -1. In practice, not all model parameters are of interest. In this case, we would first partition the information matrix and work with the submatrix corresponding to the parameters of interest.

Specifically, we first partition the design matrix $\mathbf{X} = [\mathbf{X}_1, \mathbf{X}_2]$, where $\mathbf{X}_1$ contains the columns of the design matrix pertaining to nuisance parameters and $\mathbf{X}_2$ contains columns corresponding to the parameters of interest. The vector of model parameters θ is likewise partitioned as $\theta = (\tau,\gamma)'$ or $(\tau, \gamma_s, \gamma_m)'$, representing the direct treatment effects and carryover effects. Then, with Σ denoting the covariance matrix, the information matrix can be written as

$$I_d(\theta) = X_2'\Sigma^{-1}X_2 - X_2'\Sigma^{-1}X_1\left(X_1'\Sigma^{-1}X_1\right)^{-1}X_1'\Sigma^{-1}X_2. \tag{3}$$

Following [13], a design is universally optimal if (i) its information matrix is completely symmetric, and (ii) it maximizes the trace of the information matrix. To study the universal optimality of treatment effects in the t treatments N-of-1 designs, we obtain the information matrix for the parameters of interest under the traditional model. Then the universally optimal designs could be constructed as long as the conditions given by [13] are satisfied.

2.1 Cycles and sequences

We first discuss how to find N-of-1 designs for comparing two treatments by minimizing the variance of the estimated direct treatment effect contrast, τ. To this end, it is helpful to define sequence feature parameters and show the association between them and the sequences in N-of-1 designs is useful for finding optimal N-of-1 trials for model (1) and (2) .

For N-of-1 trials involving two treatments, the design sequences consist of crossover pairs, AB and BA. Within each crossover pair, the two treatments are distinct. For two consecutive crossover pairs, the treatments assigned to the second period in the previous pair and the first period in the latter pair can be different or the same.

Further, if an AB pair is followed by a BA pair, as in $ABBA$ (or $BAAB$), we define the design as having alternating pairs in the sequence. The performance of an N-of-1 trial sequence is related to how the pairs AB and BA alternate. The following feature parameters define how AB and BA alternate in a sequence.

- s: the number of subsequences of AA and BB;
- m: the number of subsequences of AB and BA;
- $h = s - m$: the indicator of how often treatments crossed between subsequences .

When we define s and m, the subsequences can be constructed by either the treatments from a crossover pair, or be the treatments assigned to the second period in

h	s	m
$-(p-1)$	0	p-1
$-(p-3)$	1	p-2
$-(p-5)$	2	p-3
⋮	⋮	⋮
-1	$\frac{p}{2}-1$	$\frac{p}{2}$

Table 1.
Feature parameters of a sequence in a 2-treatment N-of-1 design.

h	Sequence	Alternation	*s*	*m*
−7	*ABABABAB*	0	0	7
−5	*ABABABBA*	1	1	6
	ABABBABA		1	6
	ABBABABA		1	6
−3	*ABABBAAB*	2	2	5
	ABBAABAB		2	5
	ABBABAAB		2	5
−1	*ABBAABBA*	3	3	4

Note: s = the number of AA and BB;m = the number of AB and BA in a treatment sequence, and $h = s - m$.

Table 2.
Sequences for $p = 8$ with corresponding design parameter values.

the previous pair and the first period in the latter pair. Therefore, in a p-period sequence, there are $p-1$ such subsequences with a length of 2. By the definition of feature parameters, we have $s + m = p - 1$. Determined by how a sequence is constructed, the value of h is negative and takes on possible values in $-1, -3, \cdots, -(p-1)$. **Table 1** displays the relationship among h, s and m.

For a particular h, we calculate s and m by setting $s = (p - 1 + h)/2$ and $m = (p - 1 - h)/2$. Further, for any given p, the N-of-1 designs can be classified by h. As an example, for $p = 8$, **Table 2** shows the relationship between the design sequences and the feature parameters.

In the next section, we show that the information matrix of the parameters of interest are only dependent on the feature parameters. That is, sequences with the same h values have the same information matrix. For instance, when $h = -3$, the three sequences *ABABBAAB*, *ABBAABAB*, *ABBABAAB* and their dual sequences share the same information matrix. If this h is the optimum value, the 8 period N-of-1 trials can use any of these three sequences and their duals.

3. Optimal 2-treatment N-of-1 designs

Let $\mathbf{x}_\tau$, $\mathbf{x}_\gamma$, $\mathbf{x}_s$ and $\mathbf{x}_m$ be the design vectors corresponding to the parameters τ, γ, γ_s and γ_m, respectively. Under the traditional model, the design matrix is $[\mathbf{1}_p, \mathbf{x}_\tau, \mathbf{x}_\gamma]$ for the parameters $[\mu, \tau, \gamma]$ with $\mathbf{X}_1 = 1_p$ and $\mathbf{X}_2$=$[\mathbf{x}_\tau, \mathbf{x}_\gamma]$. Under the self and mixed effect model, we have $[\mathbf{1}_p\ \mathbf{x}_\tau, \mathbf{x}_s, \mathbf{x}_m]$ for the parameters $[\mu, \tau, \gamma_s, \gamma_m]$ with $\mathbf{X}_1 = 1_p$ and $\mathbf{X}_2 = [\mathbf{x}_\tau, \mathbf{x}_s, \mathbf{x}_m]$.

In 2-treatment N-of-1 trials, the $I_d(\tau, \gamma)$ is a function of the quantities:

$$x_\tau' x_\tau = p,\ \ x_\gamma' x_\gamma = p - 1,\ \ x_\tau' x_\gamma = h \tag{4}$$

under model (1) for $\theta = (\tau, \gamma)'$, or

$$x_\tau' x_s = s,\ \ x_s' x_s = s,\ \ x_m' x_s = 0,\ \ x_\tau' x_m = -m,\ \ x_m' x_m = m \tag{5}$$

under model (2) for $\theta = (\tau, \gamma_s, \gamma_m)'$. Hence, the information matrix can be expressed in terms of p, s, m and h.

Since the information matrices can be further simply expressed in terms of h and p only, for a given p, the optimal $p-$period N-of-1 trial is completely determined by h, and much simpler to construct than previously. We proceed by defining $I_d(\tau)$ appropriately to find designs that maximize the information below.

Under an equi-correlated error assumption, the optimal N-of-1 trial for τ and γ is the one sequence design that consists of pairs of *AB* and *BA* appearing alternatively. Hence, the optimal N-of-1 trials for 4, 6, and 8 periods are the one sequence design, *ABBA*, *ABBAAB* and *ABBAABBA*, respectively. One could switch *A* and *B* to obtain a dual sequence with the same effect.

Under the equi-correlated errors, the optimal N-of-1 trial for estimating the direct treatment contrast is the sequence with only *AB* (*BA*) pairs with no alternation, such as *BABABA* and *ABABABAB*. A closed form for the optimal h is complicated for autoregressive errors, and selected numerical results are found when $h = 1 - p$.

To summarize, the optimal N-of-1 trials for estimating direct treatment effects are determined by the three feature parameters h, s, and m. However, specifying one of these along with p determines the design sequence, as illustrated in **Table 2**. We used h to summarize the optimal designs under both the traditional and self and mixed models for 4, 6, 8, 10, and 12-period N-of-1 trials.

It can be shown that under the traditional model, the optimal trial for the direct treatment effect uses the sequence with $h = -1$ for all covariance structures. Therefore, the optimal N-of-1 trial for estimating the direct treatment effect is to alternate between *AB* and *BA* pairs. In case that the carryover effect is of interest, it can be easily shown that these designs are also optimal for estimating the carryover effect, which can be obtained using the same technique for optimal designs in treatment effects. Under the self and mixed effects model, the optimal N-of-1 trial for the direct treatment effect uses a sequence with $h = -(p - 1)$ for both uncorrelated and equal-correlated covariances. Therefore, the optimal N-of-1 trial is to use only *AB* pairs throughout. Under the auto-regressive covariance structure, however, the optimal designs depend on the value of p and the auto-regressive correlation ρ. Generally, the optimal design uses *AB* and *BA* pairs alternately, but as ρ or p increases, some abnormalities are observed.

4. Optimal aggregated N-of-1 trial designs with $N > 1$

In addition to the interest in the patient-based evidence of a treatment contrast, it may also be desirable to obtain a population average effect of treatments.

Aggregating the series of N-of-1 trials can give such an estimate of the average effect [7]. Using the one sequence that was found optimal for N-of-1 trial to all patients seems to be an obvious choice. However, it might not optimize the trial for estimating the effects on the average patient and therefore, using the one sequence that is optimal for a single individual patient to all patients might not serve this purpose.

The optimal designs for aggregated N-of-1 trials can also be derived from the information matrices we obtained, similarly as for N-of-1 trials for one patient, by allowing $j = 1, \dots, N$ with $N > 1$. We approached the problem in two steps; first, we optimize single N-of-1 trials, as the primary goal is to optimize estimating the effects for each patient. Next, we optimize the overall N-of-1 trials in aggregation.

To find the optimal design, we typically choose N_k for $k = 1, \dots, s$ to allocate patients to a sequence s. The sufficient condition on N_k was given by [20] for a design to be optimal. The condition is called a duality in the design matrices, as defined earlier. Among other things, it permits simplification of the search for the optimal choice for N_k (see also [16]).

As noted earlier for **Table 1**, designs with the same value of h perform equally in estimation precision. Although all or only one of those with an equally optimal h can be used in a trial, practical consideration will lead to using the least necessary number of sequences for ease of treatment administration. Further, we found that there is a unique N-of-1 trial sequence in all p-period experiments. Since the designation of A and B is arbitrary, the optimal N-of-1 trial can be obtained by reversing the order of treatment administration. For example, the optimal 6-period N-of-1 trial is *ABBAAB* under the traditional model for $N = 1$. Its dual, *BAABBA* also has the same value of $h = -1$ and is optimal. Hence, when $N = 1$, either of these two sequences will provide the maximum amount of information. When $N > 1$ and a multiple of 2, we can adopt both of these sequences, as they maximize the information, and this approach also simplifies the search for the optimal design for estimating the treatment effect for the average patients, satisfying the duality condition in [20]. Based on this rationale, we make the following two propositions.

Proposition 1: The optimal design for aggregated N-of-1 trials under the traditional model is to allocate the same number of patients to the optimal sequence with *AB* and *BA* alternating and its dual.

For example, the optimal design for aggregated six-period N-of-1 trials is the two-sequence design using sequences *ABBAAB* and *BAABBA*, allocating the same number of patients to each. For a balanced design, N must be a multiple of 2.

Proposition 2: The optimal design for aggregated N-of-1 trials under the self and mixed model is to allocate the same number of patients to the optimal sequence with no alternation between *AB* and *BA* pairs and its dual. However, under the autocorrelation errors, the optimal design is to allocate the same number of patients to the optimal sequence that alternates between *AB* and *BA* pairs subsequently and its dual.

For example, the optimal aggregated 6-period N-of-1 trials for multi-clinic setting is to use the two-sequence design *ABABAB* and *BABABA* under the equal or uncorrelated errors, and to use the two-sequence design *ABBAAB* and *BAABBA* under the autocorrelated errors, allocating the same number of patients to each sequence.

From each sequence, we obtain individual patient specific treatment effects and by aggregating these one sequence of N-of-1 trials, we can quantify the average treatment effects.

4.1 Numerical comparisons

To appreciate the practical performance of the optimal N-of-1 trials we constructed, we compare the efficiencies of selected designs for estimating the treatment and carryover effects under the two models. We also investigate their performances in some aggregation for estimating the average treatment effect. We limit the comparison to the models with independent and equi-correlation errors. In our comparisons, we also reference many designs, labeled with an A or S at the beginning, like A65 and S83, that were investigated in [31].

Recall that the optimal N-of-1 trials are either to alternate between *AB* and *BA* pairs or simply to repeat the *AB* pair in a sequence. Under the traditional model, the optimal N-of-1 trial uses *ABBAAB* and *ABBAABBA* for 6 and 8 period experiments, respectively. We refer them to S63 and S83. Under the self and mixed effects model, the optimal N-of-1 trial is to use *ABABAB* and *ABABABAB* for 6 and 8 period experiments, respectively, which we refer to S61 and S81. **Table 3** considers other mixtures and shows that the optimal individual-based N-of-1 trials are S63 and S81 under the respective models, as expected. We also observe from the table that (i) there are no real practical differences among various N-of-1 trials under the self and mixed model, and (ii) designs S61 and S81 cannot estimate self carryover effects, making S63 and S83 preferable. Therefore, we recommend using a sequence that alternates between *AB* and *BA* pairs, such as S63 and S83, as robust and optimal N-of-1 trials for all models.

Based on these single sequence trials, we also consider aggregated N-of-1 trials to numerically justify Propositions 1 and 2. We constructed 5 aggregated N-of-1 trials for $p = 6$ and $p = 8$ with $N = 32$ and compare their efficiencies for estimating the average treatment effects as follows.

- A61. *ABABAB* and its dual with 16 patients in each sequence
- A62. *ABABBA* and its dual with 16 patients in each sequence
- A63. *ABBAAB* and its dual with 16 patients in each sequence
- A64. *ABBAAB*, *ABABBA* and their duals with 8 patients in each sequence
- A65. All 8 sequences, S61–S64 and their duals with 4 patients in each sequence
- A81. *ABABABAB* and its dual with 16 patients in each sequence
- A82. *ABABBABA* and its dual with 16 patients in each sequence
- A83. *ABBAABBA* and its dual with 16 patients in each sequence
- A84. *ABABBABA*, *ABBABAAB* and their duals with 8 patients in each sequence
- A85. All 8 sequences, S81–S84 and their duals with 4 patients in each sequence

The design A63 uses the optimal sequence S63 under the traditional model; the design A61 uses the optimal sequence S61 under the self and mixed model although the self carryover effect is not estimable; the design A62 is a slight rearrangement of

Design	h	Traditional model		Self and mixed model		
		var($\hat{\tau}$)	var($\hat{\gamma}$)	var($\hat{\tau}$)	var($\hat{\gamma}_s$)	var($\hat{\gamma}_m$)
S61: ABABAB	−5	1.208	1.500	1.208	NE	1.500
S62: ABABBA	−3	0.242	0.300	1.250	3.000	1.500
S63: ABBAAB	−1	0.173	0.214	1.214	1.714	1.714
S64: ABBABA	−3	0.242	0.300	1.250	3.000	1.500
A61 = S61 + dual		1.208	1.500	1.208	NE	1.500
A62 = S62 + dual		0.242	0.300	1.250	3.000	1.500
A63 = S63 + dual		0.173	0.214	1.214	1.714	1.714
A64 = S63 + S62 + duals		0.193	0.240	1.210	2.063	1.563
A65 = S61:S64 + duals		0.242	0.300	1.214	2.535	1.521
S81: ABABABAB	−7	1.146	1.333	1.146	NE	1.333
S82: ABABBABA	−5	0.229	0.267	1.167	2.667	1.333
S83: ABBAABBA	−1	0.127	0.148	1.150	1.600	1.400
S84: ABBABAAB	−3	0.150	0.174	1.147	1.647	1.412
A81 = S81 + dual		1.146	1.333	1.146	NE	1.333
A82 = S82 + dual		0.229	0.267	1.167	2.667	1.333
A83 = S83 + dual		0.127	0.148	1.150	1.600	1.400
A84 = S82 + S84 + dual		0.176	0.205	1.147	1.945	1.358
A85 = S81:84 + dual		0.176	0.205	1.147	1.945	1.358

Note: NE means "Not Estimable." For $N = 1$, a six-period N-of-1 trial may consider any one of S61,⋯, S64. For $N > 1$, aggregated six-period N-of-1 trials may use a combination of these, A61,⋯, A65. Similarly, an eight-period N-of-1 trial may consider any one of S81,⋯, S84. For $N > 1$, aggregated six-period N-of-1 trials may use a combination of these, A81,⋯, A85. The variances reported are divided by σ_ε^2/N (under an independence error) or $\sigma_\varepsilon^2(1-\rho)/N$ (under an equi-correlated error).

Table 3.
Variances of the estimators of treatment and carryover effects in six- and eight-period designs.

designs A61 and A63; the design A64 is a combination of designs A62 and A63; the design A65 contains all 8 possible sequences of a 6-period design. Designs A81–A85 are also similarly constructed from various N-of-1 trials. We compare these designs under the traditional model and the self and mixed model. **Table 3** displays the comparison results under the two models and reports the variances of the estimated τ, γ, γ_s and γ_m after they are divided by their leading constants σ^2/N (when errors are independent) or by $\sigma^2(1-\rho)/N$ (when errors equi-correlated).

Table 3 shows that under the traditional model, the design A63 with the optimal sequence *ABBAAB* and its dual provides the best precision for estimating both the direct treatment effect and the carryover effect for the average patients. Each of the sequences optimally estimates the individual-based treatment effect. The least efficient choice would be the design A61. Design A65, which has been used in a recent multi-clinical trial [7], is rather inefficient as well, not to mention the unnecessarily lengthy administration time and cost required to manage many treatment groups, which requires the number of patients to be a multiple of 8.

When using the self and mixed effects model, Design A61 provides the best precision for estimating the direct treatment effect and the mixed carryover effect. However, the self carryover effect is not estimable. Overall, A63 is the optimal choice even in this case. However, all designs performed rather similar with over 95% relative efficiency under the self and mixed effects model, as observed earlier for single N-of-1 trials.

A similar observation is possible for 8-period designs and their sequences. In summary, it appears that there is no discernable advantage to distinguish among the two models and various error structures.

Overall, S63 and S83 for single N-of-1 trials or designs A63 and A83 in aggregation of S63, S83 and their duals seem to be the best under both models. They are optimal for estimating direct treatment and mixed carryover effects. Further, they are optimal for estimating both the treatment and carryover effects under the traditional model. Hence, we conclude that the optimal six-period aggregated N-of-1 trials is *ABBAAB* and its dual *BAABBA*, while the optimal eight-period aggregated N-of-1 trials is *ABBAABBA* and its dual *BAABBAAB*. For an N-of-1 trial, using one of these sequences will optimize the treatment for an individual patient.

We close this section with a summary note. Our numerical work suggests that alternating *AB* and *BA* pairs in sequence is likely to result in an optimal or nearly optimal $p-$period design for all the models we have considered for estimating both individual effects in N-of-1 trials and average effects in aggregated N-of-1 trials.

5. Universally optimal N-of-1 designs for more than two treatments

Oftentimes, N-of-1 trials deal with comparing $t > 2$ treatments and we briefly discuss selected universal optimal N-of-1 trials for such a situation. In N-of-1 trials with $t > 2$ treatments, we can consider a sequence consisting of treatments in blocks of a size t. Every block within the sequence contains each of the t treatments exactly once. It follows that N-of-1 designs constructed in this way can ensure treatments are compared fairly, and poor balance can be prevented when the study is terminated prematurely. For example, in a 3-treatment N-of-1 trial, a six-period design could be *ABC*|*BCA*, where the sign | divides them into blocks. Li [31] denoted such a class of N-of-1 trial designs by No1(t,t), where the first t in the notation represents the number of treatments in the study and the second t denotes that the treatments are to be administered to be in blocks of size t. Therefore, a six-period design in the above example is No1(3,3).

Li [31] showed that Kiefer's conditions could not be satisfied with designs in the class No1(t,t). However, if we consider a slightly different class of designs, then universally optimal designs can be obtained. Li [31] used No1(t,t+) to denote the new class of designs, which consist of designs with one extra treatment to the last period in No1(t,t). For instance, a design in No1(3,3+) could be *ABC*|*BCA*|*A*, *ABC*|*BCA*|*B*, or *ABC*|*BCA*|*C*. Similarly, some examples from the class No1(2,2+) are *AB*|*BA*|*A*, *AB*|*BA*|*B*, etc.

One disadvantage of the universally optimal designs for $t > 2$ treatments is that the length of the sequence can be unmanageable, leading to drop-outs and non-compliances before the end of the trials. As discussed in [3], a universally optimal design in No1(t,t+) requires the length of the sequence equal to $(t-1)!t^2+1$, which is 5 for $t=2$, 19 for $t=3$, and 97 for $t=4$. It may be infeasible in practice because the longer the period of the experiment, the more expensive the experiment and the higher the risk of drop-outs. To shorten the length of the experiment without losing the balance in the comparison of treatments, Li [31] introduced a class of designs in No1(t,s) or No1(t,s+) for some $s < t$, especially when $s = 2$. To do so, the restriction that the block size must be equal to the number of the treatments can be relaxed [31]. By allowing the block size to be smaller than t, universally optimal designs can be manageable in practice, thereby reducing the risk of early dropouts and the burden of treatment administration.

Li [31] showed some practical universally optimal designs for three-, four- and five-treatment in blocks of size 2. In each block, two different treatments are assigned such as a crossover pair. For t-treatment designs, there are $t(t-1)$ different kinds of crossover pairs. To construct the universally optimal design, the crossover pairs are selected such that each subsequence of A_iA_j, $1 \le i, j \le t$, appears only once. Therefore, for universally optimal designs, the number of periods is $p = t^2 + 1$. For example, p is 10 for three-treatment designs, 17 for four-treatment designs and 26 for five-treatment designs. We close by giving examples of universally optimal designs in selected situations. Omitting details, which are available in [31], they are:

- No1(3,2) with $t = 3$:

$$\{ABBCCAACBA\} \quad or \quad \{BCABBAACCB\},$$

- No1(4,2+) for $t = 4$:

$$\{ABBCCDDACBDCADBAA\} \quad or \quad \{BCCDDAABBDCADBACB\}$$

and

- No1(5,2) for $t = 5$:

$$\{ABBCCDDEEAACBDCEDAEBADBECA\} \quad or$$
$$\{CDDEEAABBCCEBDACBEDBAECADC\}.$$

6. Concluding remarks

In this Chapter, we discussed and reviewed construction of universally optimal N-of-1 designs and how they may be aggregated to estimate treatment effects for the average patients. Originally, Kiefer [13] proposed the concept of universal optimality with zero row and column sums in the information matrices. We examined conditions when such universally optimal designs exist with special application to N-of-1 trial designs that will make them optimal no matter what criteria are applied. In particular, we first presented a sufficient condition that ensures N-of-1 designs are universally optimal for the traditional model that accommodates the carryover effects. Additionally, we discussed extensions of our work to finding optimal aggregated N-of-1 designs. Using numerical results from our simulation for comparing the estimated precision of several six- and eight-period designs, we were able to obtain realistic guidelines for the practitioners.

Overall, there are three key conclusions from this chapter. The first is that alternating between *AB* and *BA* pairs in sequence will result in an optimal or nearly optimal N-of-1 trial for a single patient for models considered in this chapter. In particular, our work suggests that alternating between *AB* and *BA* pairs in a single trial is quite robust to mis-specification in the error structures considered in the chapter. Consequently, there is less need to guess or conduct a pilot study to verify model assumptions and the error structures.

Another take home message is that when an experiment has been carried out with the optimal N-of-1 trial and additional patients are accrued in the trial, we can aggregate these N-of-1 trials optimally by allocating the same number of patients to its dual sequence, thereby optimizing the trial for both the individual and average patients.

Lastly, we also provided a strategy for finding N-of-1 trials with more than 2 treatments. By restricting the class of designs and utilizing each subsequence, we constructed universally optimal N-of-1 trial designs when there are $t = 3$, 4, or 5 treatments.

Author details

Yin Li[1], Weng Kee Wong[2] and Keumhee Chough Carriere[3*]

1 Ontario Medical Association, Toronto, ON, Canada

2 Department of Biostatistics, University of California-Los Angeles, LA, CA, USA

3 Department of Mathematical and Statistical Sciences, University of Alberta, Edmonton, AB, Canada

*Address all correspondence to: kccarrie@ualberta.ca

References

[1] Duan N, Kravitz R, Schmid C. Single-patient (n-of-1) trials: A pragmatic clinical decision methodology for patient-centered comparative effectiveness research. Journal of Clinical Epidemiology. 2013;**66**:S21-S28

[2] Nikles CJ, Clavarino AM, Del Mar CB. Using N-of-1 trials as a clinical tool to improve prescribing. British Journal of General Practice. 2005;**55**:175-180

[3] Scuffham PA, Nikles J, Mitchell GK, Yelland MJ, Vine N, Poulos CJ, et al. Using N-of-1 trials to improve patient management and save costs. Journal of General Internal Medicine. 2010;**25**(9): 906-913

[4] Kravitz RL, Duan N. Design and Implementation of N-of-1 Trials: A user's Guide. USA: Agency for Healthcare Research and Quality; 2014

[5] Gabler NB, Duan N, Vohra S, Kravitz RL. N-of-1 trials in the medical literature a systematic review. Medical Care. 2011;**49**:761-768

[6] Chen X, Chen P. A comparison of four methods for the analysis of N-of-1 trials. PLoS One. 2014;**9**(2): e87752

[7] Zucker DR, Ruthazer R, Schmid CH. Individual (N-of-1) trials can be combined to give population comparative treatment effect estimates: Methodologic considerations. Journal of Clinical Epidemiology. 2010;**63**: 1312-1323

[8] Punja S, Xu D, Schmidc C, Hartling L. N-of-1 trials can be aggregated to generate group mean treatment effects: A systematic review and meta-analysis. Journal of Clinical Epidemiology. 2016; **76**:65-75

[9] Li J, Gao W, Punja S, Ma B, Vohra S, Duan N, et al. Reporting quality of N-of-1 trials published between 1985 and 2013: A systematic review. Journal of Clinical Epidemiology. 2016;**76**:57-64

[10] Senior HE, Mitchell GK, Nikles J, Carmont SA, Schluter PJ, Currow DC, et al. Using aggregated single patient (N-of-1) trials to determine the effectiveness of psychostimulants to reduce fatigue in advanced cancer patients: A rationale and protocol. BMC Palliative Care. 2013;**12**(1):1-6

[11] Larson EB. N-of-1 clinical trials: A technique for improving medical therapeutics. Western Journal of Medicine. 1990;**152**:52

[12] Edgington ES. Statistics and single case analysis. Progress in Behavior Modification. 1984;**16**:83-119

[13] Kiefer J. General equivalence theory for optimum designs (approximate theory). The Annals of Statistics. 1975;**2**: 849-879

[14] Cheng CS, Wu CF. Balanced repeated measurements designs. The Annals of Statistics. 1980;**8**:1272-1283

[15] Kershner RP, Federer WT. Two-treatment crossover designs for estimating a variety of effects. Journal of the American Statistical Association. 1981;**76**:612-619

[16] Carriere KC, Reinsel GC. Investigation of dual-balanced crossover designs for two treatments. Biometrics. 1992;**48**:1157-1164

[17] Kunert J, Stufken J. Optimal crossover designs in a model with self and mixed carryover effects. Journal of

the American Statistical Association. 2002;**97**:898-906

[18] Kunert J, Stufken J. Optimal crossover designs for two treatments in the presence of mixed and self-carryover effects. Journal of the American Statistical Association. 2008;**103**: 1641-1647

[19] Carriere KC. Crossover designs for clinical trials. Statistics in Medicine. 1994;**13**:1063-1069

[20] Laska EM, Meisner M. A variational approach to optimal two-treatment crossover designs: Application to carryover-effect models. Journal of the American Statistical Association. 1985; **80**:704-710

[21] Carriere KC, Li Y, Mitchell G, Senior H. Methodological considerations for N-of-1 trials. In: The Essential Guide to N-of-1 Trials in Health. Dordrecht: Springer. 2015. pp. 67-80

[22] Guyatt GH, Heyting A, Jaeschke R, Keller J, Adachi JD, Roberts RS. N of 1 randomized trials for investigating new drugs. Controlled Clinical Trials. 1990; **11**:88-100

[23] Kunert J. Optimality of balanced uniform repeated measurements designs. The Annals of Statistics. 1984; **12**:1006-1017

[24] Afsarinejad K. Circular balanced uniform repeated measurements designs. Statistics and Probability Letters. 1988;7(3):187-189

[25] Bose M, Mukherjee B. Optimal crossover designs under a general model. Statistics & Probability Letters. 2003;**62**: 413-418

[26] Kempton RA, Ferris SJ, David O. Optimal change-over designs when carry-over effects are proportional to direct effects of treatments. Biometrika. 2001;**88**:391-399

[27] Sen M, Mukerjee R. Optimal repeated measurements designs under interaction. Journal of Statistical Planning and Inference. 1987;**17**:81-91

[28] Saha R. Repeated measurements designs. Calcutta Statistical Association Bulletin. 1983;**32**:153-168

[29] Jones B, Kunert J, Wynn HP. Information matrices for mixed effects models with applications to the optimality of repeated measurements designs. Journal of Statistical Planning and Inference. 1992;**78**:307-316

[30] Carriere KC, Reinsel GC. Optimal two-period repeated measurements designs with two or more treatments. Biometrika. 1993;**80**:924-929

[31] Li Y. Optimal Crossover Designs in Clinical Trials. Canada: University of Alberta; 2017